Milady's Standard Fundamentals for Estheticians Exam Review

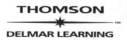

THOMSON
™
DELMAR LEARNING

Australia   Canada   Mexico   Singapore   Spain   United Kingdom   United States

NOTICE TO THE READER

Publisher does not warrant or guarantee any of the products described herein or perform any independent analysis in connection with any of the product information contained herein. Publisher does not assume, and expressly disclaims, any obligation to obtain and include information other than that provided to it by the manufacturer.

The reader is expressly warned to consider and adopt all safety precautions that might be indicated by the activities herein and to avoid all potential hazards. By following the instructions contained herein, the reader willingly assumes all risks in connection with such instructions.

The Publisher makes no representation or warranties of any kind, including but not limited to, the warranties of fitness for particular purpose or merchantability, nor are any such representations implied with respect to the material set forth herein, and the publisher takes no responsibility with respect to such material. The Publisher shall not be liable for any special, consequential, or exemplary damages resulting, in whole or in part, from the readers' use of, or reliance upon, this material.

Table of Contents

Part V - The Business of Skin Care

Foreword

Milady's Standard Fundamentals for Estheticians Exam Review has been revised to follow very closely the type of skin care questions most frequently used by states and by the national testing, conducted under the auspices of the National-Interstate Council of State Boards of Cosmetology.

This review book is designed to be of major assistance to students in preparing for the state license examinations. In addition, its regular use in the classroom will serve as an important aid in the understanding of all subjects taught in cosmetology schools and required in the practice of cosmetology.

The exclusive concentration on multiple-choice test items reflects the fact that all state board examinations and national testing examinations are confined to this type of question.

Questions on the state board examinations in different states will not be exactly like these and may not touch upon all the information covered in this review. But students who diligently study and practice their work as taught in the classroom and who use this book for test preparation and review should receive higher grades on both classroom and license examinations.

Chapter *1*

SKIN CARE HISTORY AND OPPORTUNITIES

1. Self-grooming and beautification has its origins in:
   a) the 18th century
   b) the popularity of glamorous Hollywood movies
   c) pigments that made cosmetics available to a mass audience
   d) ancient cultures, when it was often allied with the practice of medicine _____

2. Early pigments were NOT made from:
   a) minerals   c) feathers
   b) nuts   d) insects _____

3. Henna:
   a) was developed in the U.S.
   b) was first used by Hollywood makeup artist Max Factor
   c) is obtained from the powdered leaves and shoots of the mignonette tree
   d) is considered extremely dangerous by modern standards _____

4. Our words cosmetics and cosmetology come from kosmetikos, a word from what language?
   a) Egyptian   c) Latin
   b) Greek   d) Hebrew _____

5. The first modern cosmetic compound:
   a) was invented for actors and actresses in the 18th century
   b) contained highly refined petroleum
   c) was cold cream
   d) We aren't sure what the first cosmetic compound was, but we know it came from Egypt. _____

6. Fragrant oils were used in the Middle Ages:
   a) only for religious purposes
   b) as a perfume by those who could afford them
   c) Fragrant oils were not used in the Middle Ages.
   d) as hair dyes _____

7. We know about the history of cosmetic use through:
   a) its depiction in paintings
   b) its depiction in movies
   c) carbon dating
   d) DNA testing _____

8. Wigs were popular in:
   a) the age of Marie Antoinette
   b) the reign of Elizabeth I
   c) the Renaissance
   d) all of these ages _____

9. The Victorian age of the 19th century was a time:
   a) when elaborately colored clothing was common
   b) when heavy use of cosmetics on the cheeks and lips was the norm
   c) of austere and restrictive fashions and cosmetic use
   d) when headdresses were sometimes a foot tall _____

10. In the 1920s:
    a) Americans' use of cosmetics was influenced by movie stars.
    b) To imitate the look of forbidden rouge and lipstick, women pinched their cheeks and bit their lips.
    c) Eye shadow was not used.
    d) Skin, hair, and body treatment was still like that of the Victorian Age. _____

11. Because of shortages during World War II:
    a) Most women made their own cosmetics out of insects, berries, and other natural sources, often grown in Victory Gardens.
    b) Cosmetic use was banned by the government.
    c) Cosmetics were rationed.
    d) In spite of wartime shortages, sales of cosmetics and grooming aids grew. _____

12. A cosmeceutical is:
    a) any spa treatment that includes cosmetics
    b) an ancient Greek process of creating pigments
    c) a cosmetic with therapeutic properties
    d) a manicure _____

13. Which of the following are NOT contemporary "anti-aging" treatments?
    a) cosmeceuticals
    b) nutriceuticals
    c) techniceuticals
    d) neuroceuticals _____

14. Which of the following factors shaped 20th-century cosmetic use?
    a) Hollywood movies
    b) the invention of the Internet
    c) the World War II ban on cosmetics
    d) increased average lifespan _____

15. Estheticians:
    a) deal with the overall health and well-being of the skin
    b) were ancient Greek inventors of many of today's pigments
    c) are any people who use cosmetics
    d) are experts in the history of cosmetic use _____

16. Estheticians:
    a) provide care and treatment to keep the skin healthy
    b) may manufacture cosmetics
    c) detect skin problems that may require medical attention
    d) all of the above are correct _____

17. Career options for estheticians include work in:
    a) art galleries
    b) department stores
    c) police departments
    d) sports medicine _____

18. Medical esthetics:
    a) is another term for plastic surgery
    b) involves the integration of surgical procedures and aesthetic treatments
    c) is performed only by registered nurses
    d) is performed only by a physician _____

19. A medical esthetician may work in:
    a) a community health center
    b) a dermatologist's office
    c) a nursing home
    d) a morgue _____

20. A medi-spa offers:
    a) spa services and surgical procedures in a medical setting
    b) spa services and surgical procedures in a spa setting
    c) a staff of esthetician MDs
    d) Medi-spas do not exist yet under current licensing laws. _____

21. A medical esthetician does NOT need to know:
    a) basic skin care skills
    b) cosmetic chemistry
    c) organic chemistry
    d) business skills _____

22. Which of the following services is offered by a laser center?
    a. microdermabrasion   c. spider vein removal
    b. peel   d. none of the above
                                     are correct   _____

23. A make-up artist commonly works with:
    a) police officers   c) morticians
    b) soldiers   d) dentists   _____

24. Camouflage therapy is:
    a) a technique for hiding facial scarring or congenital defects
    b) a makeup technique in which cosmetic colors are blended with the
       client's natural tones
    c) a technique to help medical estheticians develop their color sense
    d) an Egyptian art involving kohl, a silver-white, metallic
       substance   _____

25. A licensed esthetician rarely:
    a) travels   c) needs business skills
    b) owns her own salon   d) none of the above
                                     are correct   _____

26. An esthetician employed as a department store salesperson might:
    a) work as a cashier
    b) sell exclusively his or her own product line
    c) produce educational books for the esthetics market
    d) travel frequently to manufacturers' showrooms   _____

27. As an esthetics educator, you would:
    a) need to meet the requirements other teachers of
       career preparations courses do
    b) need supervisory skills
    c) need to keep up with developments in the field
    d) all of the above are correct   _____

28. As an educator in the field of esthetics, you might work:
    a) for a cosmetics manufacturer
    b) for a cosmetology school
    c) to establish, amend, and repeal laws involving the industry
    d) all of the above are correct   _____

29. State licensing examiners do NOT:
    a) supervise medi-spa care
    b) ensure ethical standards are met
    c) conduct examinations
    d) enforce state regulations   _____

30. What interest can you combine with your career in esthetics?
    a) journalism   c) working with public
    b) science   d) all of the above are correct   _____

31. What factors will NOT influence esthetics in the 21st century?
    a) aging baby boomers
    b) fast-paced, stressful American lifestyles
    c) new techniques in marketing
    d) skin transplants   _____

32. Kohl is:
    a) a fragrant oil invented in the Middle Ages
    b) used as a perfume in a cosmetic related to arsenic
    c) the Greek spelling for "coal," an ancient form of eye makeup
    d) an Egyptian hair dye   _____

33. Which trend was characteristic of the 1970s?
    a) well-scrubbed look
    b) heavy eyeliner and false eyelashes
    c) individual look-your-best style
    d) platinum-blond hair   _____

34. A manufacturer's representative would:
    a) demonstrate company products
    b) work to build clientele and increase product sales
    c) visit salons
    d) all of the above are correct   _____

35. Since 1900 the average lifespan in the U.S. has:
    a) almost doubled   c) quadrupled
    b) almost tripled   d) increased only slightly   _____

Answer Key

1—d	19—b
2—c	20—a
3—c	21—c
4—b	22—c
5—c	23—c
6—b	24—a
7—a	25—d
8—d	26—a
9—c	27—d
10—a	28—d
11—d	29—a
12—c	30—d
13—d	31—c
14—a	32—c
15—a	33—c
16—d	34—d
17—b	35—a
18—b	

Chapter 2

YOUR PROFESSIONAL IMAGE

1. What is image?
   a) the way you speak and carry yourself
   b) the clothes you wear
   c) the way you relate to people
   d) all of the above are correct   _____

2. What creates a client's mental picture of you as a professional?
   a) your appearance, attitude, energy, and professional connections
   b) your appearance, attitude, abilities, and energy
   c) your appearance, personal concerns, abilities, and energy
   d) your appearance, attitude, abilities, and ability to solve their personal problems   _____

3. In addition to helping clients to look their best, what is your role?
   a) alerting them to lifestyle decisions
   b) critiquing their clothes
   c) reviewing their eating habits
   d) setting up an exercise program   _____

4. Appearance and poise are as necessary for your success as what two other traits?
   a) technical knowledge and skills
   b) skills and knowledge of the latest fashion trends
   c) technical knowledge and professional connections
   d) skills and ability to listen to people's problems   _____

5. To achieve balance, which habits should you avoid?
   a) taking drugs
   b) smoking
   c) drinking excessively
   d) all of the above are correct   _____

6. Which of these are habits does NOT help you create balance?
   a) eating a nutritious diet
   b) exercising infrequently
   c) getting adequate rest
   d) making time from work for some recreation   _____

7. One exercise session can generate up to two hours of what?
   a) relaxation response
   b) low endorphins
   c) queasiness
   d) lost time at work   _____

8. What is one of the most important aspects of personal hygiene for an esthetician?
   a) sweet-smelling fragrance
   b) nail care
   c) jewelry that will be attractive to clients
   d) sharing your makeup   _____

9. The basics of personal hygiene include which of the following?
   a) brushing your teeth instead of using mouthwash
   b) showering often enough so that underarm deodorant or antiperspirant is not necessary
   c) varying your skin care routine
   d) washing your hands when beginning a service   _____

10. Which of the following is true about your makeup?
    a) If customers admire your makeup, offer to share it with them.
    b) Makeup is a breeding ground for bacteria.
    c) For health reasons, you should continue using your makeup until it is all gone.
    d) Makeup is bacteria-free.   _____

11. Which guideline is appropriate for dress in the workplace?
    a) Uniforms should fit as loosely as possible.
    b) Women may wear high heels to complement their outfit.
    c) Hair may be worn loose and flowing to complement an outfit.
    d) Dangling jewelry is inappropriate.   _____

12. Why is good posture so important for an esthetician?
    a) It can prevent fatigue.
    b) It portrays an image of confidence.
    c) It can enhance your attractiveness.
    d) all of the above are correct   _____

13. Which is a guideline for a proper sitting posture?
    a) Keep your back straight.
    b) Cross your legs at the ankles.
    c) Always bend forward at the waist.
    d) Stand with your weight primarily on the balls of your feet.   _____

14. Which is a guideline for a proper standing posture?
    a) Keep your shoulders lifted high.
    b) Keep your knees straight in a locked position.
    c) Do not lift your upper body so that your chest is out and up.
    d) Keep your head up and chin level with the floor.   _____

15. Which is true of your conduct in the workplace?
    a) It is not as important as your appearance in determining your professional image.
    b) "Workplace conduct" refers to how you get along with your clients, coworkers, and employers.
    c) You may always express your personal feelings with clients as long as you are honest.
    d) It is unaffected by your attitude.   _____

16. What is an ingredient of a healthy, well-developed attitude?
    a) being straightforward but not critical in your dealings with others
    b) keeping all your feelings to yourself
    c) being sensitive enough to offer criticism even when it is harsh
    d) focusing solely on your own feelings and ideas, and not those of others   _____

17. Which of these workplace behaviors is considered appropriate?
    a) arriving late to work for personal reasons
    b) cleaning the treatment room, rather than leaving it for the colleague who left it messy
    c) accidentally treating a client with a substance to which they are allergic because you were unaware of the allergy
    d) not keeping abreast of current techniques because of other demands on your time   _____

18. Why is it sometimes difficult to be a team player?
    a) Both clients and employers can be demanding.
    b) It is difficult to put common goals ahead of your own.
    c) Colleagues must be dedicated to sharing the workload to alleviate stress.
    d) all of the above are correct   _____

19. What traits help make a good team?
    a) respect and caring
    c) criticizing one another
    b) focus on individual goals
    d) all of the above are correct   _____

20. Which is a good method for resolving conflict?
    a) Do not waste time getting others' opinions before making a judgment.
    b) It is better not to stand your ground.
    c) Direct a situation to a higher authority if necessary.
    d) all of the above are correct   _____

21. How can you lessen the potential for conflict?
    a) Keep to yourself as much as possible.
    b) Avoid no-win situations.
    c) Avoid interaction with different personality types.
    d) Communicate as little as possible.   _____

22. What is a good strategy for coping with a difficult client?
    a) Be friendly by informally giving personal or health advice.
    b) Just pretend to listen.
    c) Don't discuss salon rules that the client may object to.
    d) Be assertive but respectful.   _____

23. What are ethics?
    a) principles of good character, proper conduct, and a fashionable appearance
    b) principles of moral judgment and good character
    c) good time-management techniques
    d) money-earning techniques   _____

24. What are some of an esthetician's professional ethics, or principles?
    a) maintain competency
    b) act responsibly
    c) protect client confidentiality
    d) all of the above are correct   _____

25. What exemplifies integrity in the workplace?
    a) informing the client about additional services that they need, even if your employer does not offer those services
    b) borrowing a colleague's supplies to satisfy a customer's request
    c) charging a customer less than your employer's price structure calls for
    d) encouraging clients to buy your employer's products even if they may not be suitable for the client   _____

26. Who sets the ethical standards for cosmetologists?
    a) individual employers
    b) a state board
    c) the esthetician's own moral principles
    d) the clients' expectations   _____

27. Which of the following is considered to be ethical behavior?
    a) relying on a manufacturer's literature to ensure a product's efficacy
    b) socializing with clients
    c) avoiding continuing education workshops so you won't
       become too attached to a certain product or technique
    d) referring a client to another professional for a service that
       is not your expertise   _____

28. Which life skills can help in your profession?
    a) maintaining a cooperative attitude
    b) trying not to develop close friendships
    c) avoiding different situations
    d) both a and b are correct   _____

29. Which is NOT an important life skill?
    a) being genuinely caring   c) living day to day
    b) having a sense of humor   d) striving for excellence   _____

30. Which of the following is an example of a guideline for success?
    a) Let others help you define success.
    b) Tell yourself that mistakes are not okay.
    c) Avoid closing off your personal life when you are at work.
    d) Trust your ability to reach your goals.   _____

31. Which habits will help you maintain peak performance?
    a) procrastination and perfectionism
    b) self-criticism and perfectionism
    c) pacing yourself and staying productive
    d) pacing yourself and self-criticism   _____

32. Which behavior helps you come up with a game plan?
    a) just letting things happen
    b) avoiding asking yourself where you want to be in five years
    c) living from day to day
    d) determining what training you'll need to reach your goal   _____

33. What is the most important part of successful goal-setting?
    a) learning to relax when you have met your initial goals of fame and fortune
    b) having a plan and reexamining it often
    c) veering from your plan as often as possible
    d) not being concerned about whether you are staying on track _____

34. What is an example of a long-term goal?
    a) scoring a high grade on an upcoming midterm
    b) owning your own salon someday
    c) anything you can accomplish within the year
    d) reexamining your hair and makeup style _____

35. What is a good time management technique?
    a) Take on a little more than you think you can handle.
    b) Don't take time out for small rewards for yourself.
    c) Do not neglect physical activity.
    d) If you are upset, keep plowing ahead and do not take a time-out. _____

36. How should you go about prioritizing?
    a) Make a list of tasks in order of most to least important.
    b) Do not worry about taking on extra tasks that you did not count on.
    c) Don't be distracted by making schedules.
    d) all of the above are correct _____

37. What is true of deep breathing?
    a) You should breath deeply through your mouth.
    b) You should extend your abdomen outward as you inhale.
    c) It calms but does not energize.
    d) Practice it once a day at most. _____

38. What is good technique for learning punctuality in the workplace?
    a) Get a solid understanding of how long each treatment will take.
    b) Practice each treatment until the timing becomes second nature.
    c) Determine a method for maintaining an organized approach.
    d) all of the above are correct _____

39. What is a good technique for being prepared in the workplace?
    a) Clean and organize your treatment room at the beginning of the day, not at the end.
    b) Do not waste time reviewing a client's records.
    c) Do not spend time discussing retail products that the client is currently using.
    d) Allow time for follow-up or sales calls. _____

40. What is a good time-saving technique for estheticians?
    a) Decide on possible treatment procedures before the client arrives.
    b) Divide your attention between your current client and preparations for the next one.
    c) Eliminate discussion of a home care program.
    d) Make it clear that the client should not expect the treatment to be relaxing. _____

41. What should clients expect during their appointment?
    a) to fill out a client history form before the session begins
    b) to have a relaxing session
    c) to discuss a home care program
    d) all of the above are correct _____

42. Why is managing your time so important?
    a) so that you can schedule as many appointments as possible
    b) so that you will reach your goal of wealth much faster
    c) so that you can pace yourself to reach your goal
    d) so that you can stand above your colleagues _____

Answer Key

1—d	22—d
2—b	23—b
3—a	24—d
4—a	25—a
5—d	26—b
6—b	27—d
7—a	28—a
8—b	29—c
9—d	30—d
10—b	31—c
11—d	32—d
12—d	33—b
13—a	34—b
14—d	35—c
15—b	36—a
16—a	37—b
17—b	38—d
18—d	39—d
19—a	40—d
20—c	41—d
21—b	42—c

Chapter 3

SANITATION AND DISINFECTION

1. All microbes are:
   a) pathogenic
   b) microscopic
   c) parasitic
   d) viral
   _____

2. Single-celled microorganisms that cause disease are:
   a) pathogenic bacteria
   b) nonpathogenic bacteria
   c) pathogenic viruses
   d) nonpathogenic viruses
   _____

3. Streptococci cause which of the following diseases?
   a) HIV
   b) pneumonia
   c) blood poisoning
   d) colds
   _____

4. Which of the following bacteria causes syphilis?
   a) bacilli
   b) diplococci
   c) cocci
   d) spirilla
   _____

5. When bacteria is NOT active, it can:
   a) form protective spores
   b) seek out a dark damp environment
   c) divide into two cells
   d) starve from lack of sufficient food
   _____

6. Which of the following diseases is NOT caused by bacteria?
   a) anthrax
   b) syphilis
   c) HIV
   d) tetanus
   _____

7. If bacterial spores have been in an inactive stage because their living conditions have been unfavorable, they will die when conditions become
   favorable if they have been:
   a) heated to a very high temperature
   b) treated with a strong disinfectant
   c) frozen
   d) none of the above are correct   _____

8. How can one get HIV?
   a) through saliva exchanged when kissing an infected person
   b) by holding hands with an infected person who has a cut
   c) through fluids exchanged through accidental nicking with a sharp
      salon instrument
   d) through fluids exchanged through sharing beverage
      glasses with an infected person   _____

9. If a doctor discovers that a patient has an inflamed liver, the doctor might
   suspect:
   a) HIV   c) influenza
   b) hepatitis   d) polio   _____

10. The body's first line of defense against infection is:
    a) unbroken skin
    b) natural immunity
    c) bloodborne pathogens
    d) white cells that fight bacteria   _____

11. Bacteria and viruses that are carried by body fluids are called bloodborne:
    a) infections   c) white cells
    b) toxins   d) pathogens   _____

12. Which of the following is a clear indication that a client has an infection?
    a) bacteria   c) pus
    b) dead skin cells   d) inflammation   _____

13. Organisms that cannot survive without drawing their nourishment from a
    host source are called:
    a) favus   c) toxins
    b) parasites   d) scabies   _____

14. If a client appears to have head lice, the esthetician should:
    a) Advise the client to consult a physician.
    b) Clean all surfaces with pesticide.
    c) Stop treating the client.
    d) all of the above are correct   _____

15. When the bloodstream carries the bacteria or virus and their poisons to all parts of the body, the result is:
    a) a virus   c) an abscess
    b) a local infection   d) a general infection   _____

16. Molds, mildews, and yeasts are all examples of:
    a) fungi   c) vegetable bacteria
    b) animal parasites   d) skin disease   _____

17. It is important to wash your hands often during flu season because good hygiene adds to:
    a) acquired immunity   c) natural immunity
    b) acquired antibiotic   d) natural antibiotic   _____

18. Which of the following is NOT a reason to keep your salon spotlessly clean?
    a) to fill clients with confidence
    b) to create a great first impression
    c) to confidently meet vigorous health standards
    d) none of the above are correct   _____

19. Why was the Occupational Safety and Health Administration (OSHA) created?
    a) to regulate employee toxic substances and inform employees about the dangers of materials used in the workplace
    b) to ensure that clients are protected in a workplace that uses toxic materials
    c) to ensure the rights of clients to know what is contained in the products the esthetician is using
    d) to license salons and other businesses in which workers and clients might be exposed to toxins   _____

20. The highest level of decontamination is:
    a) sterilization   c) sanitation
    b) disinfection   d) none of the above
                                     are correct   _____

21. Which of the following would you do to decontaminate a lancet used to aid comedone extraction?
    a) soak in a sanitizing solution   c) heat in an autoclave
    b) wipe with disinfectant   d) wash with an antibacterial   _____

22. Which of the following cannot be cleaned in an autoclave?
    a) stainless steel lancets   c) electrolysis needles
    b) glass electrodes   d) tweezers   _____

23. Which of the following should one sterilize?
    a) countertops   c) hands
    b) lancets   d) towels   _____

24. Even strong disinfectants will NOT kill:
    a) the virus that causes HIV
    b) the virus that causes hepatitis
    c) bloodborne pathogens
    d) bacterial spores   _____

25. Disinfectants used in salons must meet standards set by:
    a) the American Academy of Dermatology
    b) the Environmental Protection Agency
    c) the American Institute of Aesthetics
    d) the Occupational Safety and Health Act   _____

26. Since it is a skin care professional's responsibility to be on constant alert for disease-causing contaminants it is important to choose a disinfectant that is:
    a) bactericidal   c) virucidal
    b) fungicidal   d) all of the above
                                                    are correct   _____

27. If tweezers you're using accidentally come into contact with a client's blood, what will you do to comply with OSHA cleaning standards?
    a) Immerse the tweezers in a bactericide.
    b) Immerse the tweezers in a tuberculocide.
    c) Wipe the tweezers with a bactericide.
    d) Wipe the tweezers with a tuberculocide.   _____

28. Quaternary ammonium compounds, or quats, are:
    a) toxic sterilizers   c) fast-acting disinfectants
    b) odorless sanitizers   d) none of the above
                                                    are correct   _____

29. To avoid softening, plastic bottles should NOT be washed in:
    a) phenols
    b) fungicides
    c) quats
    d) pseudomonacides _____

30. If isopropyl alcohol is at 65% strength, it would be a legal disinfectant:
    a) in most states
    b) in a small number of states
    c) in all states
    d) in no states _____

31. Which of the following is NOT a good safety precaution when using disinfectants?
    a) Always add water to disinfectant, not disinfectant to water.
    b) Never pour quats, phenols, alcohol, or any other disinfectant over your hands.
    c) Never place any disinfectant or other product in an unmarked container.
    d) Always wear gloves and safety glasses when mixing chemicals with water. _____

32. Disinfecting soak solution should be changed:
    a) twice a day
    b) weekly
    c) daily
    d) every other day _____

33. Instruments that are soaked in disinfectant:
    a) are cleaned by the disinfectant
    b) should be cleaned before disinfecting
    c) should be cleaned after disinfecting
    d) should be cleaned before and after disinfecting _____

34. Which of the following is NOT a recommended way to avoid recontaminating disinfected instruments?
    a) remove them from the disinfecting solution with gloves
    b) store them in a clean dry container
    c) leave them in the disinfecting solution until they are needed
    d) none of the above are correct _____

35. The contact points of electrical equipment such as electrotherapy tools:
    a) should be cleaned by immersing them as far as possible in warm soapy water
    b) do not need to be cleaned because the electricity acts as a disinfectant
    c) should be cleaned in an autoclave only
    d) should be cleaned with an EPA-registered, hospital-grade disinfectant created especially for electrical equipment _____

36. When a client's treatment is complete you must:
    a) sterilize all non-porous surfaces including door knobs and handles
    b) disinfect all non-porous surfaces including door knobs and handles
    c) sterilize all non-porous tools including your esthetic bed
    d) sanitize all non-porous tools including your esthetic bed   _____

37. In which of the following ways can you handle a disinfected product without fear of cross-contamination?
    a) with sanitized hands
    b) with gloved hands
    c) with a disinfected spatula
    d) with a spatula that has only been used on that client   _____

38. Which of the following must you do if you or your client is accidentally cut with a sharp instrument?
    a) Apply antiseptic and/or styptic without contaminating the container.
    b) Discard all disposable contaminated objects by double-bagging.
    c) Immerse all implements that have come into contact with blood or body fluids in an EPA-registered, hospital-grade disinfectant.
    d) all of the above are correct   _____

39. Allergens and pathogens can be transmitted throughout a salon if:
    a) wet rooms are not sanitized regularly
    b) air systems are not well-engineered
    c) trash can lids are opened and closed by hand rather than foot pedal
    d) sink trims and drains are not adequately sealed   _____

40. Universal precautions established by the Centers for Disease Control suggest that one should:
    a) treat the blood and bodily fluids of all clients as if it is infected
    b) ask clients if they are HIV-positive before treatment
    c) remind clients that they might have an infection even if they have no symptoms
    d) make sure that clients have been tested for HIV, hepatitis, and other bloodborne diseases   _____

Answer Key

1—b	21—c
2—a	22—b
3—c	23—b
4—d	24—d
5—a	25—b
6—c	26—d
7—d	27—b
8—c	28—c
9—b	29—a
10—a	30—d
11—d	31—a
12—c	32—c
13—b	33—b
14—d	34—c
15—d	35—d
16—a	36—b
17—c	37—c
18—d	38—d
19—a	39—b
20—a	40—a

Chapter 4

ANATOMY AND PHYSIOLOGY

1. What plays an important part in cell reproduction and metabolism?
   - a) protoplasm
   - b) cytoplasm
   - c) nucleus
   - d) muscles   _____

2. What is mitosis?
   - a) a process by which the cells are nourished
   - b) the process by which most cells reproduce
   - c) the anabolism phase of metabolism
   - d) the catabolism phase of metabolism   _____

3. What best describes metabolism?
   - a) a process by which the cells are nourished
   - b) the process by which most cells reproduce
   - c) each breathing cycle where an exchange of gases takes place
   - d) a process by which blood flows through the body   _____

4. What is NOT a primary function of the skeletal system?
   - a) provides protective covering on body surfaces
   - b) protects various organs
   - c) helps produce red and white blood cells
   - d) stores most of the body's calcium   _____

5. What removes toxic products of digestion?
   - a) kidneys
   - b) liver
   - c) lungs
   - d) small intestine   _____

6. Which system includes skin, oil, and sweat glands?
   - a) the skeletal system
   - b) the integumentary system
   - c) the circulatory system
   - d) the excretory system   _____

7. What connects two or more bones?
   a) muscle
   b) nerve fibers
   c) joint
   d) dendrites _____

8. Which bone joins all the bones of the cranium together?
   a) sphenoid bone
   b) lacrimal bones
   c) mandible bones
   d) malar bones _____

9. What kind of bones are cheekbones?
   a) ethmoid bones
   b) frontal bones
   c) occipital bones
   d) malar bones _____

10. The "Adam's apple" is what?
    a) the sternum
    b) the hyoid bone
    c) the cervical vertebrae
    d) the thorax _____

11. The humerus bone is where?
    a) the leg
    b) the palm
    c) the wrist
    d) the arm _____

12. What is true about the insertion part of the muscle?
    a) Pressure in massage usually begins there.
    b) It is the immovable part of the muscle.
    c) It is the middle part of the muscle.
    d) It is the hole in the muscle. _____

13. Which muscle causes wrinkles across the forehead?
    a) aponeurosis
    b) frontalis
    c) occipitalis
    d) epicranius _____

14. Which body part has muscles that are nonfunctioning?
    a) ear
    b) eyebrow
    c) nose
    d) chin _____

15. A function of the orbicularis oculi muscle is to:
    a) close the eye
    b) lower the jaw
    c) rotate the head
    d) draw the eyebrow down _____

16. A function of the mentalis muscle is to:
    a) help you smile
    b) wrinkle your chin
    c) pull down the mouth
    d) elevate the lip _____

17. A function of the trapezius muscle is to:
    a) shape the mouth
    b) pucker the lips
    c) swing the arms
    d) assist in breathing
    _____

18. The biceps are where?
    a) front and inner side of the upper arm
    b) front and outer side of the upper arm
    c) back of the lower arm
    d) back of the upper arm
    _____

19. A function of the flexor muscles is to:
    a) turn the palm
    b) bend the wrist
    c) straighten the wrist
    d) rotate the palm
    _____

20. Which muscles cover the shoulder joint?
    a) pronator muscles
    b) supinator muscles
    c) deltoid muscle
    d) pectoralis major and serratus anterior muscles
    _____

21. Which system provides the physical foundation of the body?
    a) the circulatory system
    b) the muscular system
    c) the nervous system
    d) the skeletal system
    _____

22. The brain, spinal cord, and nerves are part of what system?
    a) the circulatory system
    b) the muscular system
    c) the nervous system
    d) the skeletal system
    _____

23. Which system controls the five senses?
    a) the circulatory system
    b) the muscular system
    c) the nervous system
    d) the skeletal system
    _____

24. The brain is:
    a) a muscle
    b) nerve tissue
    c) glands
    d) capillaries
    _____

25. What controls sensation and glandular activity?
    a) the heart
    b) the brain
    c) the spinal cord
    d) the eyes
    _____

26. Where does the spinal cord begin?
    a) the back
    b) the brain
    c) the shoulders
    d) the neck
    _____

27. The cell body and nucleus, dendrites, and an axon make up what?
    a) muscles
    c) glands
    b) tissues
    d) nerve cell
    _____

28. What receives impulses from other neurons?
    a) nucleus
    c) axon
    b) dendrites
    d) veins
    _____

29. What transmits impulses that produce reactions to elements such as heat and cold?
    a) motor nerves
    c) sensory nerves
    b) veins
    d) spinal column
    _____

30. Which nerve supplies the arm and hand?
    a) ulnar
    c) fifth cranial
    b) median
    d) radial
    _____

31. Which nerve is in the little finger?
    a) ulnar
    c) fifth cranial
    b) median
    d) radial
    _____

32. The infratrochlear nerve affects what area?
    a) the muscles of the upper cheek
    b) the skin between the eyes and nose
    c) the membrane and skin of the nose
    d) the side of the nose, upper lip, and mouth
    _____

33. The seventh cranial is a:
    a) motor nerve
    c) bone
    b) sensory nerve
    d) skull
    _____

34. Which nerve controls chewing?
    a) ulnar
    c) fifth cranial
    b) median
    d) radial
    _____

35. The buccal nerve affects what?
    a) the muscles of the mouth
    b) the side of the neck
    c) the muscles of the chin and lower lip
    d) the eyebrow
    _____

36. The temporal nerve affects what?
    a) the muscles of the mouth   c) the chin and lower lip
    b) the side of the neck   d) the eyebrow   _____

37. The cervical nerves affect what?
    a) the chest
    b) the scalp at the front of the head
    c) the face and forehead
    d) the scalp at the back of the head and neck   _____

38. Which nerve is located at the base of the skull?
    a) the smaller occipital nerve   c) the greater auricular nerve
    b) the greater occipital nerve   d) the radial nerve   _____

39. Which nerve supplies the thumb?
    a) the smaller occipital nerve   c) the greater auricular nerve
    b) the greater occipital nerve   d) the radial nerve   _____

40. What does the digital nerve supply?
    a) the knee   c) the fingers
    b) the toes   d) the eyebrow   _____

41. What part of the body does the radial nerve and its branches supply?
    a) the upper arm and "funny bone" elbow
    b) the foot, the side of the leg, and the back of the knee
    c) the thumb, the side of the arm, and the back of the hand
    d) the face and the back of the skull   _____

42. Which system coordinates all other systems?
    a) circulatory system   c) endocrine system
    b) digestive system   d) nervous system   _____

43. Which is a function of lymph?
    a) controls the circulation of the blood
    b) carries food and nourishment to the cells
    c) carries waste and impurities from the cells
    d) helps cell reproduction   _____

44. The heart is what shape?
    a) kidney   c) cone
    b) circle   d) diamond   _____

45. A main function of the vagus nerve is to:
    a) supply the muscles of the scalp
    b) supply the muscles of the face
    c) regulate the heartbeat
    d) supply the muscles of the lower abdomen   _____

46. The vagus nerve is also known as the:
    a) fifth cranial   c) tenth cranial
    b) seventh cranial   d) medial   _____

47. What best describes the ventricles?
    a) the thin-walled chambers of the heart
    b) the lower, thick-walled chambers of the heart
    c) the membranes which enclose the heart
    d) the valves that allow blood to flow in one direction   _____

48. Which type of circulation sends blood from the heart to the lungs?
    a) pulmonary   c) general
    b) systemic   d) none of the above
                                    are correct   _____

49. What best describes the atrium?
    a) a thin-walled chamber of the heart
    b) a lower, thick-walled chamber of the heart
    c) the membrane which encloses the heart
    d) a valve that allows blood to flow in one direction   _____

50. Veins carry blood containing:
    a) oxygen   c) waste products
    b) hormones   d) nourishment   _____

51. Which statement is NOT a true statement about blood?
    a) Blood carries water, oxygen, and food to the cells of the body.
    b) Blood is bright red in the veins and dark red in the arteries.
    c) Blood carries carbon dioxide and waste products to
       be eliminated.
    d) Blood helps equalize the body's temperature.   _____

52. What best describes blood?
    a) nutritive fluid in body
    b) an average body contains approximately 6-8 pints
    c) circulates through the nervous system
    d) sticky and sweet   _____

53. What are the components of blood?
    a) platelets, plasma, and hemoglobin
    b) red corpuscles, platelets, plasma, and hemoglobin
    c) white corpuscles, platelets, plasma, and hemoglobin
    d) red and white corpuscles, platelets, plasma, and hemoglobin _____

54. What best describes hemoglobin?
    a) 90 percent water
    b) main function is to carry food and secretions to the cells
    c) complex iron protein
    d) destroys disease-causing germs _____

55. What is a main function of plasma?
    a) contributes to blood clotting
    b) takes carbon dioxide away from body cells
    c) carries oxygen to the body cells
    d) destroys disease-causing germs _____

56. What is a main function of platelets?
    a) contributes to blood clotting
    b) takes carbon dioxide away from body cells
    c) carries oxygen to the body cells
    d) destroys disease-causing germs _____

57. What is a main function of white blood cells?
    a) contributes to blood clotting
    b) takes carbon dioxide away from body cells
    c) carries oxygen to the body cells
    d) destroys disease-causing germs _____

58. Red blood cells contain:
    a) platelets   c) hemoglobin
    b) white blood cells   d) plasma _____

59. Which system acts as an aid to the blood system?
    a) muscular system   c) lymph vascular system
    b) integumentary system   d) skeletal system _____

60. Which statement does NOT describe the lymph vascular system?
    a) carries nourishment from the body to the body cells
    b) affects the growth and development of the body
    c) removes waste material from the body cells
    d) provides a suitable fluid environment for the cells _____

61. The facial artery supplies blood to where?
    a) lower region of the face
    b) upper region of the face
    c) top of the head and scalp
    d) back of the head _____

62. The common carotid arteries supply blood to:
    a) the brain
    b) the head
    c) the scalp
    d) the neck _____

63. The internal carotid arteries supply blood to:
    a) the brain
    b) the head
    c) the scalp
    d) the neck _____

64. The submental artery supplies what?
    a) blood to the chin
    b) blood to the lower lip
    c) blood to the side of the nose
    d) blood to the upper lip _____

65. The superior labial artery supplies what?
    a) blood to the chin
    b) blood to the lower lip
    c) blood to the side of the nose
    d) blood to the upper lip _____

66. What does the inferior labial artery supply?
    a) blood to the chin
    b) blood to the lower lip
    c) blood to the side of the nose
    d) blood to the upper lip _____

67. The angular artery supplies what?
    a) blood to the chin
    b) blood to the lower lip
    c) blood to the side of the nose
    d) blood to the upper lip _____

68. The parietal artery is a branch of what artery?
    a) the frontal artery
    b) the superficial temporal artery
    c) the transverse facial artery
    d) the middle temporal artery _____

69. What does the posterior auricular supply?
    a) blood to the scalp and ear area
    b) blood to the back of the head
    c) blood to the front of the ear
    d) blood to the upper eyelid _____

70. Which artery supplies blood to the front of the ear?
    a) the anterior auricular artery   c) the transverse facial artery
    b) the angular artery   d) the middle temporal artery   _____

71. The internal and external jugular veins carry:
    a) blood returning to the heart from the arms
    b) blood returning to the head from the heart
    c) blood returning to the heart from the head
    d) blood returning to the heart from the legs   _____

72. What best describes the endocrine system?
    a) controls the steady circulation of blood
    b) affects the growth, development, and health of the body
    c) purifies the body by the elimination of waste
    d) protective covering that helps regulate the body's temperature   _____

73. What removes certain elements from the blood to convert them into new compounds?
    a) glands   c) capillaries
    b) arteries   d) veins   _____

74. What do exocrine glands produce?
    a) sweat   c) insulin
    b) estrogen   d) adrenaline   _____

75. What are the two main types of glands?
    a) exocrine and radial   c) radial and median
    b) endocrine and radial   d) exocrine and endocrine   _____

76. Which statement best describes the digestive system?
    a) eliminates waste material
    b) changes food into nutrients and waste
    c) produces sweat
    d) transports food through the bloodstream   _____

77. A main function of digestive enzymes is to:
    a) secrete hormones directly into the blood stream
    b) eliminate waste matter
    c) metabolize various toxic substances
    d) change food into a form that can be used by the body   _____

78. Which statement best describes the excretory system?
    a) eliminates waste material
    b) changes food into nutrients and waste
    c) produces sweat
    d) transports food through the bloodstream   _____

79. A main function of the kidneys is to:
    a) eliminate perspiration   c) eliminate decomposed food
    b) discharge bile   d) excrete urine   _____

80. A main function of the liver is to:
    a) eliminate perspiration   c) eliminate decomposed food
    b) discharge bile   d) excrete urine   _____

81. A main function of the large intestine is to:
    a) eliminate perspiration   c) eliminate decomposed food
    b) discharge bile   d) excrete urine   _____

82. The respiratory system consists of what?
    a) heart and lungs   c) kidneys, liver, and large
                                        intestine
    b) lungs and air passages   d) skin, hair and nails   _____

83. Which best describes the diaphragm?
    a) muscular wall that separates the thorax from the abdominal region
    b) thin wall that separates the thorax from the abdominal region
    c) muscular wall that separates the heart from the lungs
    d) thin wall that separates the heart from the lungs   _____

84. During inhalation, or breathing in, what is absorbed into the blood?
    a) carbon monoxide   c) oxygen
    b) carbon dioxide   d) none of the above
                                        are correct   _____

85. Which statement best describes the integumentary system?
    a) eliminates waste material
    b) changes food into nutrients and waste
    c) includes hair and nails
    d) transports food through the bloodstream   _____

Answer Key

1—c	44—c
2—b	45—c
3—a	46—c
4—a	47—b
5—b	48—a
6—b	49—a
7—c	50—c
8—a	51—b
9—d	52—a
10—b	53—d
11—d	54—c
12—a	55—b
13—b	56—a
14—a	57—d
15—a	58—c
16—b	59—c
17—c	60—b
18—a	61—a
19—b	62—b
20—c	63—a
21—d	64—a
22—c	65—d
23—c	66—b
24—b	67—c
25—b	68—b
26—b	69—a
27—d	70—a
28—b	71—c
29—c	72—b
30—b	73—a
31—a	74—a
32—c	75—d
33—a	76—b
34—c	77—d
35—a	78—a
36—d	79—d
37—d	80—b
38—a	81—c
39—d	82—a
40—c	83—a
41—c	84—c
42—d	85—c
43—c	

Chapter 5

CHEMISTRY FOR ESTHETICIANS

1. All cosmetic creams, lotions, and masks are made of:
   a) surfactants
   b) plants
   c) chemicals
   d) synthetics
   _____

2. The two branches of chemistry are:
   a) synthetic and esthetic
   b) laboratory and natural
   c) organic and inorganic
   d) There are more than two branches of chemistry.
   _____

3. Inorganic substances:
   a) burn easily
   b) are carbon-rich chemicals
   c) include some categories of plants
   d) are not and never were alive
   _____

4. The three different states of matter are:
   a) organic, inorganic, and carbon
   b) space, property, and form
   c) solid, liquid, and gas
   d) There are only two states of matter.
   _____

5. Matter can be classified into what three main groups?
   a) elements, compounds, and mixtures
   b) organic, inorganic, and synthetic
   c) solid, liquid, and carbon
   d) periodic, nonperiodic, and elemental
   _____

6. A molecule is formed by:
   a) joining two or more atoms chemically
   b) joining an organic with an inorganic substance
   c) joining a mixture with a compound
   d) joining a compound with an element   _____

7. Compounds and mixtures are:
   a) combinations of matter
   b) categories on the Periodic Table of Elements
   c) the two states of matter
   d) the result of chemical reactions   _____

8. We can identify matter through its:
   a) organic and inorganic compounds
   b) compounds and mixtures
   c) physical and chemical properties
   d) three states   _____

9. Chemical properties of matter:
   a) are the only way to identify matter
   b) can only be determined with a chemical reaction
   c) can be determined without a chemical reaction
   d) are organically determined   _____

10. Matter can be changed:
    a) only chemically
    b) physically and chemically
    c) through compounds and mixtures
    d) into any of its five states   _____

11. Hydrogen, nitrogen, and oxygen:
    a) can combine with other elements to form compounds
    b) can combine with other elements to form atoms
    c) are organic compounds
    d) are inorganic compounds   _____

12. The most commonly used cosmetic ingredient is:
    a) nitrogen
    b) water
    c) acid
    d) oxygen   _____

13. Hydrogen peroxide:
    a) can be used as an antiseptic and hair-lightening agent
    b) is the most commonly used ingredient in cosmetics
    c) is a suspension
    d) is an element   _____

14. pH:
    a) is the relative degree of acidity or alkalinity of a substance
    b) determines the degree of compound in a mixture
    c) determines the degree of suspension in a solution
    d) determines the amount of hydrogen per element _____

15. The acid mantle:
    a) is a barrier on the surface of the skin formed by sebum and sweat
    b) determines a compound's pH
    c) is determined by its alkali
    d) allows molecules to form compounds beneath the skin _____

16. pH adjusters or buffers in skin care products:
    a) protect the skin   c) cause irritation
    b) dissolve the acid mantle   d) are always highly alkaline _____

17. A chemical reaction:
    a) can only occur in a suspension
    b) produces pH
    c) occurs when two or more chemicals are mixed together
    d) creates an acid mantle _____

18. Oxidation:
    a) is an oxidation-reduction reaction
    b) is a pH adjuster
    c) is the only way to penetrate the acid mantle
    d) reduces heat _____

19. An oxidizing agent:
    a) creates oxygen   c) destroys oxygen
    b) releases oxygen   d) reduces oxygen _____

20. What is redox?
    a) a pH buffer
    b) a contraction for reduction-oxidation
    c) an oxidizing agent
    d) a popular brand of litmus paper used by estheticians _____

21. Any cosmetic may be:
    a) a solvent, an insolvent, or an insoluble
    b) a soluble, an insoluble, or an inculcation
    c) a solution, a suspension, or an emulsion
    d) a redox, a litmus, or an alkali _____

22. A solution is a:
    a) lipophilic mixture of two or more substances
    b) hydrophilic
    c) chemical compound
    d) blended mixture of two or more substances _____

23. Miscible liquids:
    a) are high in alkali
    b) exist only in suspensions
    c) are mutually soluble
    d) are chemical compounds _____

24. A suspension is:
    a) a state in which solid particles are distributed throughout a liquid medium
    b) a blended mixture of two or more substances
    c) a substance that dissolves another substance to form a solution
    d) always an emulsion _____

25. An emulsion is:
    a) an emulsifier
    b) a mixture of two or more immiscible substances united with the aid of a binder or emulsifier
    c) a blended mixture of two or more substances
    d) a state in which solid particles are distributed throughout a liquid medium _____

26. Surfactants:
    a) are always hydrophilic
    b) are always lipophilic
    c) are never present in emulsions
    d) act as a bridge to allow substances to emulsify _____

27. A surfactant molecule has two parts, which are:
    a) hydrophobic and lipophobic
    b) hydrophilic and lipophilic
    c) hydroponic and lipoponic
    d) hydrosuction and liposuction _____

28. Modern synthetic surfactants:
    a) are highly alkaline
    b) can coat and dull the hair
    c) can form an insoluble film
    d) are superior to traditional soaps _____

29 Almost all skin care products are:
    a) oil and water emulsions
    b) oil and water solutions
    c) oil-free emulsions
    d) lipophilic solutions   _____

30. Suntan lotion is:
    a) a water-in-oil emulsion
    b) an oil-in-water emulsion
    c) a water-in-oil solution
    d) an oil-in-water solution   _____

31. Once the water and the active ingredients in an emulsion separate:
    a) the emulsion has become a solution
    b) the product is ready for use
    c) the product should be discarded
    d) Water and active ingredients do not separate in an emulsion.   _____

32. An acid is:
    a) a substance with a pH above 7.0
    b) a substance with a pH below 7.0
    c) an emulsion with a pH above 7.0
    d) an emulsion with a pH below 7.0   _____

Answer Key

1—c	17—c
2—c	18—a
3—d	19—b
4—c	20—b
5—a	21—c
6—a	22—d
7—a	23—c
8—c	24—a
9—b	25—b
10—b	26—d
11—a	27—b
12—b	28—d
13—a	29—a
14—a	30—b
15—a	31—c
16—a	32—b

Chapter 6

COSMETIC CHEMISTRY

1. What do the active agents in facial products do?
   a) cleanse and moisturize
   b) treat and cleanse
   c) normalize and moisturize
   d) all of the above are correct _____

2. Because estheticians are not yet allowed to claim the actual benefits of some products, what should you do?
   a) remain unfamiliar with them
   b) understand them
   c) claim benefits that you're sure of
   d) claim benefits that you've heard of _____

3. What distinguishes between drugs and cosmetics?
   a) the Food and Drug Administration
   b) state licensing boards
   c) the Cosmetic Act of 1938
   d) where you buy them _____

4. What is the definition of drugs?
   a) articles applied to the human body for cleansing, beautifying, promoting attractiveness, or altering the appearance
   b) products intended to affect the structures and/or function of the body
   c) products intended to affect the function of your brain
   d) products intended to improve the skin's health and appearance _____

5. What are the two accepted types of ingredients?
   a) functional and performance
   b) hydrating and cleansing
   c) cleansing and performance
   d) functional and moisturizing _____

6. Which of these tasks is NOT performed by performance ingredients?
   a) giving products body and texture
   b) hydrating the skin's surface
   c) helping patch the skin's barrier
   d) causing actual changes in the appearance of the skin   _____

7. What do alphahydroxy acids do?
   a) hydrate the skin's surface   c) help patch the skin's barrier
   b) help products spread   d) exfoliate the corneum   _____

8. Emollients are almost always:
   a) anhydrous   c) minerals
   b) fatty agents   d) powders   _____

9. What does it mean if a product is anhydrous?
   a) It does not contain any water.
   b) It can act as a performance ingredient or as a vehicle.
   c) It is nonreactive and biologically inert.
   d) It prevents dehydration.   _____

10. Oils vary in:
    a) fat content, heaviness, and color
    b) color, smell, and density
    c) density, fat content, and heaviness
    d) density, heaviness, and silicone content   _____

11. What does it mean if an oil is "biologically inert?"
    a) The oil does not react with chemicals involved in the skin's function.
    b) The oil prevents dehydration by trapping moisture.
    c) The oil does not harbor bacteria and other organisms.
    d) The oil is produced from fatty acids and alcohols.   _____

12. Which is one of the fattiest and heaviest oils?
    a) safflower   c) canola
    b) coconut   d) octyl palmitate   _____

13. Which lubricant ingredients are produced by plant oils or animal fats?
    a) silicone   c) fatty esters
    b) fatty acids   d) surfactants   _____

14. What are fatty alcohols?
    a) fatty esters that have been occluded
    b) fatty esters that have been exposed to stearic acid
    c) fatty acids that have been exposed to comedones
    d) fatty acids that have been exposed to hydrogen   _____

15. What is NOT true of silicones?
    a) They act as vehicles in products, including makeup foundation.
    b) They allow oxygen in and out of the follicles.
    c) They help trap moisture in the skin.
    d) Their names almost always end in "ate."   _____

16. What is the term for the tendency of any topical substance to cause or worsen a buildup of dead cells?
    a) hydration   c) comedogenicity
    b) aromatherapy   d) surface tension   _____

17. What is the task of a surfactant?
    a) trap the skin's moisture
    b) exfoliate dead cells
    c) reduce surface tension between the skin and the product
    d) produce sebum   _____

18. Without emulsifiers, what would oil and water do?
    a) separate into layers   c) thicken into a gel
    b) blend in a product   d) foam   _____

19. What does it mean if a substance is called oil soluble?
    a) It is mixed into the water phase of the product.
    b) It is mixed into the oil phase of the product.
    c) It is mixed into the oil and water phases of the product.
    d) It washes off with oil-based cleanser.   _____

20. What is the task of a carbomer?
    a) protects products from chemical changes
    b) reduces surface tension
    c) inhibits bacteria growth
    d) thickens creams   _____

21. Which oils can be used to relax or stimulate a client's mood?
    a) synthetic   c) essential
    b) petrolatum   d) mineral   _____

22. What prevents bacteria from living in a product?
    a) preservatives
    b) liposomes
    c) polymers
    d) betahydroxy acids   _____

23. What is the task of an antioxidant?
    a) inhibit oxidation
    b) inhibit reaction promoted by oxygen or peroxides
    c) help products retain their properties
    d) all of the above are correct   _____

24. What do metal salts do?
    a) season food
    b) provide intense color
    c) cause car rust
    d) none of the above are correct   _____

25. How many certified colors are there?
    a) 5
    b) 35
    c) 70
    d) 2   _____

26. Which colors are noncertified?
    a) yellow, blue, red
    b) zinc oxide, iron oxide
    c) inorganic
    d) orange, green   _____

27. What is NOT true of exfoliators?
    a) They can work through chemical reactions.
    b) They remove dead corneum cells.
    c) They improve the symptoms of dehydration.
    d) They knock dead cells off the skin's surface.   _____

28. Which of the following is true?
    a) Creams have more emollients than lotions or fluids do.
    b) Fluids have more emollients than lotions or creams do.
    c) Lotions have more emollients than fluids or creams do.
    d) Creams have more emollients than humectants do.   _____

29. Which of the following is responsible for most of a product's cosmetic effects?
    a) carbomers
    b) antioxidants (inhibit oxidation or reactions promoted by oxygen)
    c) talc and pigment
    d) color agents   _____

30. Which kind of technique is a delivery system?
    a) natural
    b) mechanical
    c) chemical
    d) none of the above
       are correct

    _____

31. What are some of the ingredients transferred by liposomes?
    a) hydrators
    b) antioxidants
    c) alphahydroxy acids
    d) all of the above
       are correct

    _____

32. How can the appearance of aging be slowed?
    a) by lowering oxygen intake in the cells
    b) by faciliating cell turnover with nutrients
    c) by dissolving collagen
    d) by slowing metabolic processes

    _____

33. Which high-tech ingredients stimulate metabolism?
    a) polyglucans and glycoproteins
    b) polyglucans and tissue respiratory factor
    c) glycoproteins and coenzyme Q10
    d) TRF and coenzyme Q10

    _____

34. Which ingredient derived from yeast helps reduce the appearance of fine lines and wrinkles by stimulating the formation of collagen?
    a) beta-glucans
    b) tissue respiratory factor
    c) polyglucans
    d) glycoproteins

    _____

35. What is used as the base for a setting mask?
    a) alphahydroxy acid
    b) oils derived from the earth
    c) clays derived from the earth
    d) oils derived from plants

    _____

36. When should a serum or intensive corrector be used?
    a) immediately (professional ampoules are intended for immediate one-time use)
    b) day and night for 30 to 60 days or more
    c) day and night for a week
    d) daily for one year

    _____

37. Which statement regarding absorbing sunscreen ingredients is NOT true?
    a) They neutralize UV rays.
    b) They absorb UV rays.
    c) They may be combined with particulate sunscreens in one product.
    d) Their other official name is chemical sunscreens.   _____

38. Which makeup product has a solvent base, such as mineral spirits, to make it water-resistant?
    a) eye shadow   c) lipstick
    b) eyeliner pencil   d) oil-free foundation   _____

39. If a client has an allergic reaction that requires medical treatment, when is the manufacturer responsible?
    a) if the product was sold in bulk, repackaged in smaller containers, and resold
    b) if the product was made in the salon
    c) if the product was not property labeled
    d) if a client neglected to read the label   _____

Answer Key

1—d	21—c
2—b	22—a
3—c	23—d
4—b	24—b
5—a	25—b
6—a	26—b
7—d	27—c
8—b	28—a
9—a	29—d
10—c	30—c
11—a	31—d
12—b	32—b
13—b	33—a
14—d	34—a
15—d	35—c
16—c	36—b
17—c	37—d
18—a	38—a
19—b	39—c
20—d	

Chapter 7

BASICS OF ELECTRICITY

1. Electricity is a flow of:
   - a) positively charged particles
   - b) electrons
   - c) matter
   - d) neutrons

   _____

2. Copper is a particularly good:
   - a) insulator
   - b) conductor
   - c) rectifier
   - d) converter

   _____

3. What is an insulator?
   - a) a substance that does not easily transmit electricity
   - b) a material, substance, or medium that easily transmits electricity
   - c) a substance that repels
   - d) an agent that slows or interferes with a chemical action

   _____

4. Which of the following appliances is powered by direct current (DC)?
   - a) curling iron
   - b) hair dryer
   - c) flashlight
   - d) towel warmer

   _____

5. Alternating current (DC) is a(n):
   - a) rapid and interrupted current that flows first in one direction and then in the opposite direction
   - b) constant, even-flowing current that travels in one direction only and produces a chemical reaction
   - c) alternating and interrupted current that produces a mechanical eaction without a chemical effect
   - d) constant current having a positive and negative pole

   _____

6. A volt measures:
   a) the number of electrons flowing through a wire
   b) how much electric energy is used in one second
   c) the pressure or force of an electric current
   d) the resistance of an electric current.　　_____

7. An apparatus that changes direct current (DC) to alternating current (AC) is called a(n):
   a) rectifier　　　　　　　　　c) converter
   b) polarity changer　　　　　d) alternator　　_____

8. A higher amp rating indicates:
   a) higher pressure
   b) higher resistance
   c) a greater number of electrons and a stronger current
   d) a greater amount of electric energy used in a second　　_____

9. A unit that measures the amount of electricity used in one second is a(n):
   a) milliampere　　　　　　　c) wavelength
   b) watt　　　　　　　　　　d) electric current　　_____

10. Which of the following statements about electrical appliances is true?
    a) They carry energy through space on waves.
    b) They use direct current.
    c) They have a single electrical connection.
    d) They have two electrical connections.　　_____

11. An electrical plug with one rectangular prong that is larger than the other ensures good:
    a) polarity　　　　　　　　c) grounding
    b) modality　　　　　　　　d) fusing　　_____

12. Current will NOT flow through a conductor unless its force is stronger than the:
    a) amps　　　　　　　　　c) ohms
    b) watts　　　　　　　　　d) volts　　_____

13. A fuse:
    a) prevents excessive current from passing through a circuit
    b) regulates the strength of the current used
    c) measures the rate of flow of an electric current
    d) reverses the direction of an electric current from
       negative to positive　　_____

14. What is a rheostat?
    a) a device that reverses the direction of an electric current from negative to positive
    b) a switch that automatically interrupts an overloaded electric current
    c) a device that regulates the strength of the current used
    d) a device that measures the rate of flow of an electric current   _____

15. Grounding:
    a) carries current safely to the ground
    b) determines the polarity of an electric current
    c) is a way to ensure that a circuit does not become overloaded
    d) reverses the direction of an electrical current   _____

16. The Underwriter's Laboratory certification ensures the:
    a) correct polarity of an electrical appliance
    b) safety of an electrical appliance
    c) proper grounding of an electrical appliance
    d) correct amperage of an electrical appliance   _____

17. Which of the following terms refers to a modality?
    a) static electricity   c) direct current
    b) electromagnetic radiation   d) faradic current   _____

18. An anode is usually marked:
    a) blue   c) black
    b) green   d) red   _____

19. A cathode:
    a) closes the pores   c) softens tissues
    b) decreases blood supply   d) contracts blood vessels   _____

20. Polarity refers to:
    a) a type of current used in facial and scalp treatments
    b) the tendency of a battery to attract or repel
    c) direct or indirect application of high-frequency current
    d) the two main kinds of electric current   _____

21. Electrotherapy is applied with the use of a(n):
    a) wall switch   c) electrode
    b) converter   d) jack   _____

22. The most commonly used modality is:
    a) faradic current
    b) alternating current
    c) direct current
    d) galvanic current   _____

23. Never administer electrical treatments to a client with:
    a) broken capillaries
    b) pustular acne
    c) hardened sebum
    d) high blood pressure   _____

24. What is the name of the process used to soften and emulsify oil and blackheads in hair follicles?
    a) desincrustation
    b) anaphoresis
    c) microdermabrasion
    d) cataphoresis   _____

25. Sinusoidal current is best suited for use with:
    a) a person who has high blood pressure
    b) someone who has pustular skin conditions
    c) a person who has gold-filled teeth
    d) a nervous client   _____

26. Which of the following statements about Tesla high-frequency current is true?
    a) It is a light therapy that produces little heat.
    b) It is a thermal or heat-producing current.
    c) It is a good process for product penetration.
    d) It is a process that produces muscle contractions.   _____

27. Radiant energy is also known as:
    a) electricity
    b) magnetism
    c) electromagnetic radiation
    d) the visible spectrum   _____

28. Visible light makes up what percentage of natural sunlight?
    a) 10 percent
    b) 35 percent
    c) 65 percent
    d) 80 percent   _____

29. If a wavelength has low frequency it has:
    a) short waves
    b) a low number of waves
    c) a short distance between peaks
    d) short peaks   _____

30. Within the visible spectrum of light:
    a) Red has the shortest wavelength.
    b) Red has the longest wavelength.
    c) Violet has the shortest peaks between waves.
    d) Violet has the longest peaks between waves.   _____

31. Ultraviolet (UV) rays should be applied at a distance of:
    a) 6 to 10 inches   c) 20 to 24 inches
    b) 12 to 18 inches   d) 30 to 36 inches   _____

32. What type of light therapy penetrates the deepest?
    a) ultraviolet light   c) white light
    b) infrared   d) blue light   _____

Answer Key

1—b	17—d
2—b	18—d
3—a	19—c
4—c	20—b
5—a	21—c
6—c	22—d
7—c	23—d
8—c	24—a
9—b	25—d
10—d	26—b
11—c	27—c
12—c	28—c
13—a	29—b
14—c	30—b
15—a	31—d
16—b	32—b

Chapter 8

PHYSIOLOGY AND HISTOLOGY OF THE SKIN

1. What is the name for the study of the functions of the skin?
   a) histology
   b) esthetics
   c) cosmetology
   d) physiology   _____

2. What does "esthetics" refer to?
   a) the field of skin care, including waxing and makeup
   b) the field of skin care, including massage
   c) the study of the structure of the skin
   d) the integumentary system   _____

3. What does the "integumentary" system refer to?
   a) reproduction
   b) skin
   c) circulation
   d) digestion   _____

4. Which part of the body has the thinnest skin?
   a) soles of the feet
   b) ear lobes
   c) eyelids
   d) palms of the hands   _____

5. Each inch of skin contains:
   a) 15 feet of blood vessels
   b) 650 sweat glands
   c) 100 oil glands
   d) all of the above are correct   _____

6. How does massage lower stress in the body?
   a) by sending messages to the brain through nerve stimulation
   b) by tightening muscles
   c) by increasing circulation
   d) by warming the body's temperature   _____

7. How does injured skin restore itself to normal thickness?
   a) by trapping water in the outermost layer
   b) by increasing production of sebum
   c) through a hyperproduction of cells and bloodclotting ability
   d) by increasing production of melanin _____

8. What do the sensory nerve endings respond to?
   a) touch and pain   c) pressure
   b) cold and heat   d) all of the above are correct _____

9. Which of these statements is true?
   a) The body's internal thermostat changes when the outside temperature changes.
   b) The body's internal thermostat is set at 98.6 degrees Fahrenheit.
   c) Even on a very hot day, our internal temperature is not affected.
   d) none of the above are correct _____

10. How does oil help maintain the water level in the cells?
    a) Oil discharges carbon dioxide.
    b) Oil coating the skin's surface slows down water evaporation.
    c) Oil blocks the absorption of oxygen.
    d) Oil acts as intercellular cement. _____

11. When the skin breathes, what does it absorb?
    a) carbon dioxide   c) oxygen
    b) hydrogen   d) carbon monoxide _____

12. What surrounds the cells in the epidermis?
    a) lipids   c) follicles
    b) basal cells   d) prickly spine appendages _____

13. In what layer of the skin does cell division occur continuously?
    a) stratum corneum   c) basal cell layer
    b) reticular layer   d) horny layer _____

14. What passes through the stratum lucidum?
    a) blood vessels   c) oil
    b) keratin   d) light _____

15. Where is the stratum lucidum found?
    a) forehead and cheekbones
    b) eyelids and earlobes
    c) palms of hands and soles of feet
    d) toes and fingers
    _____

16. The dermis is how many times thicker than the epidermis?
    a) two times
    b) 25 times
    c) ten times
    d) 50 times
    _____

17. Which layer connects the dermis to the epidermis?
    a) reticular
    b) papillary
    c) subcutaneous
    d) stratum lucidum
    _____

18. What makes up 70% of the dermis?
    a) collagen
    b) elastin
    c) adipose
    d) keratin
    _____

19. What happens to the subcutis layer as you age?
    a) It becomes extremely dry.
    b) It is overcome with adipose.
    c) It plumps up.
    d) It decreases.
    _____

20. Which of these does the body NOT replace naturally?
    a) elastin
    b) skin
    c) bones
    d) liver
    _____

21. Which fibers are dispersed to sweat and oil glands?
    a) sensory nerve fibers
    b) motor nerve fibers
    c) secretory nerve fibers
    d) collagen
    _____

22. Where are pigment granules produced?
    a) hair follicles
    b) melanocytes
    c) eccrine glands
    d) apocrine glands
    _____

23. Which is true of sebaceous glands?
    a) If their ducts become clogged, melanin is formed.
    b) Sebaceous glands are smaller on the face and scalp.
    c) Their glandular sacs open into the hair follicles.
    d) They produce sweat.
    _____

24. When are eccrine glands more active?
    a) during physical activity
    b) during emotional changes
    c) when ducts are clogged
    d) when there is a biological reaction to potential mates
    _____

25. What causes approximately 80 to 85 percent of our aging?
    a) our skin care routine   c) the environment
    b) heredity   d) the sun's rays   _____

26. What is designed to protect the skin from the sun, but can be destroyed by large doses of UV light?
    a) melanin   c) accrine glands
    b) keratin   d) vitamin A   _____

27. Advise clients to wear protective lotion with a sunscreen of at least:
    a) SPF 1   c) SPF 40
    b) SPF 15   d) SPF 5   _____

28. When checking existing moles, what changes should you look for?
    a) asymmetry and border   c) color and diameter
    b) border and color   d) all of the above are correct   _____

29. In the American Cancer Society's ABCD checklist, what does B stand for?
    a) bloody   c) border
    b) blotchy   d) bacteria   _____

30. How does nicotine age the skin?
    a) It causes capillary walls to burst.
    b) It causes dryness and allergic reactions on the skin's surface.
    c) It contracts blood vessels, which weakens circulation and deprives tissues of oxygen.
    d) It causes a buildup of dead cells.   _____

31. How do weakened blood vessels affect the skin?
    a) They decrease circulation, depriving tissues of oxygen.
    b) They hamper healthy cell growth and secretion of dead cells.
    c) They decrease circulation, enabling a buildup of clogged pores.
    d) They weaken capillary walls, causing them to burst.   _____

32. Usually, the damage done by smoking and drinking alcohol is:
    a) easy to reverse or diminish
    b) impossible to reverse or diminish
    c) minimal
    d) hard to reverse or diminish   _____

33. What does healthy skin begin with?
    a) exercise   c) regular facials
    b) diet and water intake   d) moisturizer   _____

34. Which vitamin is also known as ascorbic acid?
    a) C   c) D
    b) A   d) E   _____

35. Vitamin A is well-known for treating which skin condition?
    a) flakiness   c) scarring
    b) burst blood vessels   d) acne   _____

36. Which vitamin is an antioxidant that can help prevent certain types of cancer?
    a) D   c) E
    b) C   d) A   _____

37. Water composes what percentage of the body's weight?
    a) 10 to 30 percent   c) 50 to 70 percent
    b) 30 to 50 percent   d) 10 to 20 percent   _____

38. What formula helps determine how many 8-ounce glasses of water you need every day?
    a) Divide your body weight by 8.
    b) Divide your body weight by 2; divide this number by 8.
    c) Divide your body weight by 4; divide this number by 8.
    d) Divide your body weight by 2; divide this number by 4.   _____

39. What is the number-one cause of daytime fatigue?
    a) lack of sleep   c) lack of water
    b) lack of exercise   d) lack of vitamin A   _____

40. All the necessary motors and parts to run our bodies are contained in:
    a) the foods we take in
    b) the water we take in
    c) the environment surrounding us
    d) chemicals our bodies produce   _____

41. What are two of the three basic food groups?
    a) proteins and vitamins   c) proteins and water
    b) carbohydrates and water   d) proteins and carbohydrates _____

42. What are enzymes?
    a) chains of essential amino acid molecules
    b) Retin A lotions
    c) catalysts that break down complex food molecules to smaller molecules
    d) catalysts that break down basic chemical sugars into simple sugars   _____

43. What is NOT one of protein's tasks?
    a) help with body growth
    b) provide energy needed for muscular work
    c) make keratin in skin, nails, and hair
    d) help with duplication of DNA   _____

44. How does the immune system use proteins?
    a) Proteins regulate the body temperature during an infection.
    b) Proteins do the infection-fighting.
    c) Proteins send white blood cells to kill the invader.
    d) Proteins define what is an invader and how the body will react. _____

45. What is included in a vegan diet?
    a) dairy products, but neither fish nor meat
    b) dairy products and fish, but no meat
    c) plant products and no dairy products
    d) meat but no dairy products   _____

46. Why is glucose the most important carbohydrate?
    a) It provides most of the body's energy.
    b) It is the chief storage form of carbohydrates in plants.
    c) It helps push waste out of the colon.
    d) It is present in skin, nails, and hair.   _____

47. What are three basic types of carbohydrates?
    a) simple sugars, starches, and fiber/cellulose
    b) complex carbohydrates, simple sugars, and starches
    c) fiber/cellulose, complex sugars, and polysaccharides
    d) polysaccharides, mucopolysaccharides, and disaccharides _____

48. What is a disaccharide made of?
    a) one molecular sugar unit   c) two molecular fiber units
    b) two molecular sugar units   d) four starch units   _____

49. Which of these are simple carbohydrates?
    a) milk and fruit sugars
    c) cereals and pastas
    b) dairy and fish
    d) honey and some vegetables _____

50. Where is glucose stored?
    a) papillary layer
    c) muscles and liver
    b) heart and blood
    d) blood and lymph   _____

51. Which foods are high in fiber?
    a) grain brans and meat
    c) cereals and dairy
    b) corn and flour products
    d) carrots and beans   _____

52. What does your body use to manufacture fat?
    a) existing fat and protein
    c) existing fat and water
    b) carbohydrates and proteins
    d) carbohydrates and water _____

53. What is the main fat in foods?
    a) triglycerides
    c) cholesterol
    b) lipids
    d) saccharides   _____

54. What do sebaceous glands use to lubricate skin?
    a) lipids
    c) ascorbic acid
    b) water
    d) lymph   _____

55. How many extra calories does it take for the body to store one
    pound of fat?
    a) 2,000
    c) 1,000
    b) 5,000
    d) 3,500   _____

56. According to many dieticians, what percentage of a person's
    entire caloric intake should be from fat?
    a) less than 20%
    c) less than 30%
    b) less than 10%
    d) less than 5%   _____

57. What is cholesterol used for?
    a) creating omega-3 fatty acids
    b) creating adipose tissue
    c) fighting cardiovascular diseases
    d) strengthening cell membranes   _____

58. Which is a source of omega-3 fatty acids?
    a) corn oil   c) dairy
    b) fish   d) beef   _____

59. Where are fat-soluble vitamins stored?
    a) liver and adipose tissue
    b) epidermis and adipose tissue
    c) liver and epidermis
    d) adipose tissue and muscles   _____

60. What are vitamins required for?
    a) breaking down and reconstructing proteins
    b) synthesizing fatty acids
    c) converting amino acids
    d) all of the above are correct   _____

61. What does "fortified" mean?
    a) Vitamin A has been added to the food product.
    b) Provitamins have been added to the food product.
    c) Vitamin C has been added to the food product.
    d) Water-soluble vitamins have been added to the product.   _____

62. Which vitamin is necessary for proper eyesight?
    a) C   c) A
    b) thiamine   d) B12

63. What is NOT a good source of vitamin D?
    a) fish oils   c) fortified milk
    b) plants   d) butter   _____

64. Which two are antioxidants?
    a) vitamin D and vitamin E   c) vitamin E and betacarotene
    b) vitamin K and betacarotene   d) vitamin B6 and B12   _____

65. Where is vitamin K found?
    a) beans   c) whole-wheat products
    b) clams   d) nuts   _____

66. Which of these is NOT a B vitamin?
    a) niacin   c) thiamine
    b) riboflavin   d) betacarotene   _____

67. What are other names for vitamins B1 and B2?
    a) thiamine and tocopherol
    b) thiamine and riboflavin
    c) niacin and biotin
    d) sunshine vitamin and riboflavin   _____

68. Enzymes that function in the energy production by cells are called:
    a) folic acid   c) amino acids
    b) riboflavin   d) niacin   _____

69. Which vitamin is strongly connected to protein synthesis?
    a) B6   c) B1
    b) B12   d) B   _____

70. Which vitamin is produced in the intestinal tract by microbes?
    a) niacin   c) biotin
    b) pyridoxine   d) folic acid   _____

71. Which two substances synthesized by pantothenic acid make up
    part of the barrier function of skin?
    a) phospholipids and folic acid
    b) hormones and cholesterol
    c) hormones and cobalamin
    d) cholesterol and phospholipids   _____

72. What can easily deplete a body's vitamin C?
    a) smoking and drug use
    b) smoking and lack of exercise
    c) smoking and stress
    d) smoking and alcohol consumption   _____

73. What vitamin should you take to combat a cold?
    a) C   c) B12
    b) K   d) D   _____

74. What inorganic materials are required for many reactions of the
    cells and the body?
    a) enzymes   c) simple sugars
    b) trace minerals   d) lipids   _____

75. A body needs only trace amounts of which minerals?
    a) magnesium and phosphorus   c) potassium and sodium
    b) iron and iodine   d) calcium and iron   _____

76. Which factors affect the amount of nutrition a body needs?
    a) age and gender
    b) gender and size
    c) pregnancy and lactation
    d) all of the above are correct _____

77. Carbohydrates should make up what percentage of the daily diet?
    a) 60 to 70 percent
    b) 20 to 25 percent
    c) 55 to 60 percent
    d) 30 to 40 percent _____

78. What happens if a woman's body fat drops too low?
    a) She loses protein in the keratinocytes.
    b) She loses muscle tissue.
    c) She has trouble synthesizing simple sugars.
    d) She has hormonal imbalances. _____

79. Which is true?
    a) Vitamins and supplements are not substitutes for proper nutrition.
    b) Vitamins and mineral supplements have good nutritional value.
    c) The best way to start a diet is to cleanse the body by fasting.
    d) If you lower your calorie intake enough, exercise is not necessary for losing weight. _____

80. In order to be effective, how should minerals be taken in?
    a) as supplements
    b) as food
    c) as topical agents
    d) as liquids _____

Answer Key

1—d	41—d
2—a	42—c
3—b	43—b
4—c	44—d
5—d	45—c
6—a	46—a
7—c	47—a
8—d	48—b
9—b	49—d
10—b	50—c
11—c	51—d
12—a	52—b
13—c	53—a
14—d	54—a
15—c	55—d
16—b	56—c
17—b	57—d
18—a	58—b
19—d	59—a
20—a	60—d
21—c	61—a
22—b	62—c
23—c	63—b
24—a	64—c
25—d	65—a
26—a	66—d
27—d	67—b
28—b	68—b
29—c	69—a
30—c	70—c
31—a	71—d
32—d	72—c
33—b	73—a
34—a	74—b
35—d	75—b
36—d	76—d
37—c	77—c
38—b	78—d
39—c	79—a
40—a	80—b

Chapter **9**

SKIN DISORDERS AND DISEASES

1. Dermatology is:
   a) the study of cosmetics manufacture
   b) the field studied by estheticians
   c) the name of a particularly malignant cyst
   d) the branch of medical science that treats the skin and its
      disorders and diseases   _____

2. Recognizing skin diseases and disorders is important for both you and
   your clients because:
   a) You will be diagnosing and treating all of their skin disorders
      and diseases.
   b) You must know what abnormalities require referral to a physician.
   c) You must take special precautions when treating infectious diseases.
   d) You do not need to know and recognize skin diseases
      and disorders.   _____

3. Any mark, symptom, or abnormality of the skin is described as:
   a) dermatology   c) a lipophile
   b) carcinoma   d) a lesion   _____

4. Primary lesions include:
   a) pimples, freckles, and mosquito bites
   b) tertiary and vascular lesions
   c) scabs, scars, and dandruff
   d) all dermatological conditions   _____

5. Bullae and vesicles are:
   a) pus-filled papules, known as pustules
   b) blisters containing clear, watery fluid
   c) tumors
   d) two types of secondary lesion   _____

6. A freckle is a type of:
   a) secondary lesion
   b) pustule
   c) macule
   d) bulla

   _____

7. A pustule is:
   a) a type of secondary lesion
   b) an example of anhidrosis
   c) an inflamed macule
   d) an inflamed, pus-filled papule

   _____

8. A tumor is:
   a) always cancerous
   b) the same as a macule
   c) an abnormal swelling varying in size, shape, and color
   d) a flat spot or discoloration on the skin

   _____

9. Poison ivy and poison oak produce:
   a) vesicles
   b) macules
   c) seborrhea
   d) rosacea

   _____

10. Secondary lesions always:
    a) develop in later stages of disease
    b) form because of infection
    c) are disorders of the sebaceous glands
    d) begin as macules

    _____

11. Dead cells that form over a wound or blemish while it's healing are known as:
    a) steatoma
    b) macules
    c) fissures
    d) crust

    _____

12. A keloid is a kind of:
    a) macule
    b) scab
    c) fissure
    d) scar

    _____

13. Acne, furnacles, and rosacea are examples of:
    a) sebaceous (oil) gland disorders
    b) sudoriferous (sweat) gland disorders
    c) pigmentation disorders
    d) the three different kinds of macule

    _____

14. Which of the following do NOT form in a hair follicle?
    a) open comedones
    b) furnacles
    c) milia
    d) blackheads

    _____

15. Rosacea is aggravated by:
    a) all spa treatments—always refer clients to dermatologists
    b) caffeine
    c) bland foods
    d) lack of exposure to sun   _____

16. Secondary lesions associated with excess oil include:
    a) macules   c) asteatosis
    b) seborrhea   d) keloids   _____

17. Masses of sebum can form:
    a) asteatosis   c) macules
    b) steatoma   d) rosacea   _____

18. Disorders of the sudoriferous (sweat) glands include:
    a) rosacea   c) prickly heat
    b) freckles   d) acne   _____

19. Excessive perspiration is called:
    a) anhidrosis   c) bromhidrosis
    b) hyperhidrosis   d) psoriasis   _____

20. Inflammations of the skin include:
    a) herpes simplex   c) vitiligo
    b) macules   d) keloids   _____

21. Contact dermatitis:
    a) is an allergic reaction
    b) is contagious
    c) can be treated but not prevented
    d) only occurs in individuals with asthma   _____

22. Eczema:
    a) always results in dry lesions
    b) always results in moist lesions
    c) can produce dry or moist lesions
    d) does not produce lesions   _____

23. Erythema is:
    a) swelling caused by injury or infection
    b) redness caused by inflammation
    c) a light, abnormal patch of skin
    d) foul-smelling perspiration   _____

24. Herpes simplex is:
    a) contagious
    b) not contagious
    c) an allergic reaction
    d) a pigment disorder _____

25. Psoriasis is:
    a) an acne-like condition around the mouth
    b) a non-contagious skin disease characterized by red patches with white-silver scales
    c) a contagious skin disease characterized by red patches with white-silver scales
    d) a recurring viral infection _____

26. Dyschromia is:
    a) a swelling caused by injury or infection
    b) abnormal pigmentation
    c) contagious
    d) a painful itching disease of the skin _____

27. Abnormal pigmentation can be caused by:
    a) only internal factors
    b) only external factors
    c) internal and external factors
    d) We don't know what causes abnormal pigmentation. _____

28. The types of dyschromia are:
    a) sebaceous and sudoriferous
    b) anhidrosis and hyperhidrosis
    c) hyperpigmentation and hypopigmentation
    d) contagious and noncontagious _____

29. Freckles, moles, and tans are examples of:
    a) keratomas
    b) leukodermas
    c) hypopigmentation
    d) hyperpigmentation _____

30. A nevus is NOT:
    a) a birthmark
    b) a mole
    c) an inflammation
    d) a port-wine stain _____

31. Albinism and vitiligo are examples of:
    a) hypoallergens
    b) hypertrophies
    c) hyperpigmentation
    d) hypopigmentation _____

32. A hypertrophy is a(n):
    a) dry, itchy patch of skin
    b) swelling caused by injury or infection
    c) abnormal growth
    d) area lacking melanin   _____

33. Abnormally thick buildups of cells are:
    a) moles   c) verrucas
    b) keratoses   d) furnacles   _____

34. Actinic keratoses are:
    a) pink or flesh-colored precancerous lesions that feel sharp or rough
    b) hypertrophies caused by a virus
    c) redness and bumpiness in the cheeks or upper arms from
       blocked follicles
    d) large blisters containing watery fluid   _____

35. Hairs in moles:
    a) are a sign of cancer and should be removed
    b) are a sign of skin tags and should not be removed
    c) are common and should not be removed
    d) are benign and should be removed by a physician   _____

36. The types of skin cancer caused by cumulative sun exposure are:
    a) hyperpigmentation and hypopigmentation
    b) basal cell carcinoma, squamous cell carcinoma, and malignant
       melanoma
    c) primary, secondary, and tertiary
    d) benign cell carcinoma, sebaceous cell carcinoma, and
       malingering melanoma   _____

37. Basal cell carcinoma:
    a) often appears as light, pearly nodules
    b) is characterized by scaly red papules or nodules
    c) is characterized by black or dark patches
    d) is undetectable   _____

38. Basal cell carcinoma is:
    a) the most common and least severe type of skin cancer
    b) normal and shouldn't be referred to a physician
    c) the most serious form of skin cancer
    d) infectious   _____

39. An example of a contagious skin disorder is:
    a) basal cell carcinoma
    c) albinism
    b) herpes simplex
    d) squamous cell carcinoma _____

40. In regards to herpes simplex, it's important to know a client's health history because:
    a) Herpes simplex is contagious even when lesions are not present.
    b) Peels, waxing, or other stimuli may cause the skin to break out even if the disease is not currently active.
    c) Herpes simplex, if left untreated, can become malignant melanoma.
    d) A client's health history is private; do not pry into this subject. _____

41. Tinea are:
    a) the first sign of a herpes outbreak
    b) the first sign of skin cancer
    c) fungal infections that estheticians routinely treat
    d) fungal infections that estheticians do not treat _____

42. Acne is:
    a) a hereditary trait
    b) a contagious virus
    c) a fungal infection
    d) an acquired, thickened patch of epidermis _____

43. Which of the following is NOT a cause of acne?
    a) bacteria
    c) clogged pores
    b) viruses
    d) stress _____

44. Clogged pores can be caused by:
    a) follicles
    c) retention hyperkeratosis
    b) hyperpigmentation
    d) macules _____

45. If a client's acne is infectious:
    a) Treat the area with caution.
    b) Refer the client to a physician.
    c) Test the area so you can diagnose the infection.
    d) There is no such thing as infectious acne. _____

46. Open and closed comedones:
    a) always result in acne problems
    b) result in acne problems if not treated
    c) are unrelated types of lesions
    d) are used to treat acne problems _____

47. Acne outbreaks include:
    a) comedones, papules, and pustules
    b) comedones, bullae, and nodules
    c) bullae, vesicles, and macules
    d) chloasma, metasma, and dyschromia   _____

48. Cystic acne:
    a) is routinely treated by estheticians
    b) can only be treated by a physician
    c) can be treated by either estheticians or physicians
    d) cannot be treated   _____

49. Comedogenic ingredients in products:
    a) are useful in treating acne
    b) can aggravate acne
    c) have no effect on acne
    d) should only be used by physicians   _____

50. A client with acne:
    a) should be treated like all other clients
    b) should use water-based products when possible
    c) should use oil-based products when possible
    d) must be referred to a physician   _____

51. Male hormones:
    a) cause a decrease in oil production and help fight acne
    b) stimulate sebaceous glands and can cause acne
    c) stimulate sudoriferous glands and can cause acne
    d) have nothing to do with acne   _____

52. Adult acne is more common in males because:
    a) Testosterone inhibits the development of acne.
    b) Testosterone contributes to the development of acne.
    c) Estrogen contributes to the development of acne.
    d) Adult acne is more common in females.   _____

53. Stress can trigger acne because:
    a) It decreases sebum production.
    b) It increases sebum production.
    c) It decreases adrenaline.
    d) It stabilizes hormonal levels.   _____

54. Certain foods:
    a) trigger acne and should be avoided
    b) may trigger acne outbreaks indirectly
    c) have high water contents and can trigger acne outbreaks
    d) Food does not affect acne.   _____

55. Acne triggers include:
    a) close contact with someone having an acne outbreak
    b) skin irritation from touching the face
    c) basal cell carcinomas
    d) dyschromia   _____

56. Grade I of acne is:
    a) the least serious   c) infectious
    b) the most serious   d) untreatable   _____

57. Acne excoriee is:
    a) the least serious form of acne
    b) the most serious form of acne
    c) the same as cystic acne
    d) a disorder where clients purposely scrape off acne lesions   _____

Answer Key

1—d	30—c
2—b	31—d
3—d	32—c
4—a	33—b
5—b	34—a
6—c	35—d
7—d	36—b
8—c	37—a
9—a	38—a
10—a	39—b
11—d	40—b
12—d	41—d
13—a	42—a
14—c	43—b
15—b	44—c
16—b	45—d
17—b	46—b
18—c	47—a
19—b	48—b
20—a	49—b
21—a	50—b
22—c	51—b
23—b	52—d
24—a	53—b
25—b	54—b
26—b	55—b
27—c	56—a
28—c	57—d
29—d	

Chapter *10*

SKIN ANALYSIS

1. What is NOT included in an in-depth skin analysis?
   a) the consultation
   b) health screening questions
   c) personal notes about the client
   d) the client chart _____

2. Skin type is based primarily upon:
   a) how old the person is
   b) how well-hydrated the skin is
   c) how much oil is produced in the skin
   d) how fair or dark the skin is _____

3. The T-Zone includes the forehead as well as:
   a) the cheeks and chin
   b) the eyes and nose
   c) the eyes and chin
   d) the nose and chin _____

4. What happens to our skin as we age?
   a) It is more likely to dehydrate.
   b) Sun damage becomes less apparent.
   c) Our oil production slows down.
   d) It becomes more sensitive. _____

5. Which skin type is usually free of blemishes?
   a) oily
   b) normal
   c) combination
   d) dry _____

6. What are antioxidants?
   a) acne breakouts after puberty
   b) free radical scavengers, vitamins, and ingredients
   c) skin lacking in oxygen
   d) acid used to exfoliate the face _____

7. Dry skin typically has pores that:
   a) are large
   b) are small
   c) change from larger to medium outside the T-Zone
   d) change from medium to smaller outside the T-Zone   _____

8. Oily skin typically has pores that:
   a) are large
   b) are small
   c) change from larger to medium outside the T-Zone
   d) change from medium to smaller outside the T-Zone   _____

9. Normal skin typically has pores that:
   a) are large
   b) are small
   c) change from larger to medium outside the T-Zone
   d) change from medium to smaller outside the T-Zone   _____

10. Combination skin typically has pores that:
    a) are large
    b) are small
    c) change from larger to medium outside the T-Zone
    d) change from medium to smaller outside the T-Zone   _____

11. Which skin type doesn't have enough sebum production?
    a) oily   c) dehydrated
    b) normal   d) dry   _____

12. Which skin type typically requires more cleansing and exfoliating?
    a) oily   c) combination
    b) normal   d) dry   _____

13. Dry skin care typically requires what type of products?
    a) exfoliating   c) maintenance
    b) water-based   d) occlusive   _____

14. Oily skin care typically requires what type of products?
    a) exfoliating   c) maintenance
    b) keratosis   d) occlusive   _____

15. Which skin type contains the most melanin?
    a) Type VI – Black   c) Type IV – Mediterranean
    b) Type V – Mideastern   d) Type I – Very fair   _____

16. Normal skin care typically requires what type of products?
    a) exfoliating   c) maintenance
    b) water-based   d) occlusive   _____

17. Which skin type is generally more sensitive and reactive?
    a) Type VI – Black   c) Type IV – Mediterranean
    b) Type V – Mideastern   d) Type I – Very fair   _____

18. What skin types have more trouble with hyperpigmention?
    a) darker skin types   c) older skin
    b) lighter skin types   d) medium skin types   _____

19. What is a sign of sensitive skin?
    a) dryness   c) redness
    b) large pores   d) acne   _____

20. Which skin type rarely burns, and always tans?
    a) Type VI – Black   c) Type IV – Mediterranean
    b) Type V – Mideastern   d) Type I – Very fair   _____

21. What does the Fitzpatrick Scale measure?
    a) the amount of dryness in the skin
    b) the amount of oil in the skin
    c) the results of stressful stimulants on the skin
    d) the skin's ability to tolerate sun exposure   _____

22. Which skin type is more prone to hypertrophic scarring?
    a) Type VI – Black   c) Type IV – Mediterranean
    b) Type V – Mideastern   d) Type I – Very fair   _____

23. Which ethnic skin type is typically one of the most sensitive?
    a) Black   c) Asian
    b) Hispanic   d) Native American   _____

24. Which ethnic skin type has the most sun protection?
    a) Black
    b) Hispanic
    c) Asian
    d) Native American
    _____

25. What are papules?
    a) blackheads and clogged pores
    b) whiteheads
    c) sagging, loose skin
    d) raised lesions/blemishes
    _____

26. Which best describes hyperpigmentation?
    a) redness caused by inflammation
    b) fluid infections under the skin
    c) white, colorless areas
    d) brown discoloration from melanin production
    _____

27. Which best describes hypopigmentation?
    a) redness caused by inflammation
    b) fluid infections under the skin
    c) white, colorless areas
    d) brown discoloration from melanin production
    _____

28. Which best describes erythema?
    a) redness caused by inflammation
    b) fluid infections under the skin
    c) white, colorless areas
    d) brown discoloration from melanin production
    _____

29. Smoking causes what condition in the skin?
    a) dehydration
    b) asphyxiation
    c) erythema
    d) papules
    _____

30. What causes up to 80% of extrinsic skin aging?
    a) smoking
    b) environmental stresses
    c) sun exposure
    d) misuse of products
    _____

31. What products protect the skin and hold in moisture?
    a) melanin
    b) alpha-hydroxy acids
    c) antioxidants
    d) occlusive
    _____

32. What is a contraindication?
    a) a buildup of cells characterized by a rough texture
    b) a scale used to measure the skin type's ability to tolerate sun exposure
    c) a skin or medical condition that could cause a treatment to have negative effects
    d) free radical scavengers, vitamins, and ingredients _____

33. What is keratosis?
    a) a buildup of cells characterized by a rough texture
    b) a scale used to measure the skin type's ability to tolerate sun exposure
    c) a skin or medical condition that could cause a treatment to have negative affects
    d) free radical scavengers, vitamins, and ingredients _____

34. What is couperous?
    a) treatments that could cause negative side affects to those with certain medical conditions
    b) distended capillaries from weakening capillary walls
    c) an excessive buildup of dead skin cells
    d) oiliness of the skin _____

35. What is milia?
    a) oil and dead skin cells trapped beneath the surface of the skin
    b) a buildup of cells characterized by a rough texture
    c) clogged pores caused by a buildup of debris
    d) acid used to exfoliate the skin _____

36. What is the preferable first step to analyzing the skin?
    a) touch and massage
    b) looking with a magnifying lamp/light
    c) looking with a Wood's lamp
    d) cleansing the skin _____

37. What products are used to exfoliate the skin?
    a) melanin   c) antioxidants
    b) alpha-hydroxy acids   d) occlusive _____

38. What best describes hyperkeratinization?
    a) distended capillaries from weakening capillary walls
    b) oiliness of the skin
    c) damage caused by sun exposure
    d) an excessive buildup of dead skin cells _____

39. What best describes seborrhea?
    a) distended capillaries from weakening capillary walls
    b) oiliness of the skin
    c) damage caused by sun exposure
    d) an excessive buildup of dead skin cells   _____

40. What is actinic skin damage caused by?
    a) sun exposure   c) misuse of products
    b) acne   d) medical conditions   _____

Answer Key

1—c	21—d
2—c	22—a
3—d	23—c
4—c	24—a
5—b	25—d
6—b	26—d
7—b	27—c
8—a	28—a
9—d	29—b
10—c	30—c
11—d	31—d
12—a	32—c
13—d	33—a
14—a	34—b
15—a	35—a
16—c	36—b
17—d	37—b
18—a	38—d
19—c	39—b
20—c	40—a

Chapter *11*

PRODUCT SELECTION AND INGREDIENTS

1. It is important to educate a client about:
   a) what a product will do for them
   b) how effective a product is
   c) how a product works
   d) all of the above are correct

   _____

2. Which of the products listed is NOT used in a facial?
   a) exfoliant
   b) Retin-A
   c) toner
   d) clay mask

   _____

3. Cleansers are recommended if they:
   a) leave a film on the skin
   b) rinse clean with water
   c) are harsh on the skin
   d) are alkaline

   _____

4. Bar soaps are ideal for daily cleaning, except they tend to:
   a) not rinse off completely
   b) leave the skin feeling oily
   c) dry out after too few washings
   d) leave the skin too tight

   _____

5. Cleansers do NOT:
   a) dissolve dirt and makeup
   b) soften the skin
   c) restore the pH balance of the skin
   d) unblock pores

   _____

6. Certain ingredients in cleansers can help many skin conditions, but cleansers CANNOT help:
   a) sensitivity
   b) dehydration
   c) capillary problems
   d) alkalinity _____

7. Which one of these products is NOT in the same product category as the others?
   a) cleansers
   b) toners
   c) fresheners
   d) astringents _____

8. Which of the following is NOT a characteristic of astringents?
   a) They help oily conditions.
   b) They fight acne.
   c) They replenish moisture.
   d) They use alcohol to remove excess oil. _____

9. Which product removes residue left behind by cleansers?
   a) exfoliant
   b) herb
   c) toner
   d) paraffin _____

10. Exfoliation treatments can include:
    a) lanolin
    b) zinc oxide
    c) alpha-hydroxy acids (AHAs)
    d) potassium hydroxide _____

11. The esthetician's domain is:
    a) the live layers of skin
    b) hygiene
    c) muscles and joints
    d) the superficial epidermis _____

12. Removal of dry, dead surface cells benefits the skin by doing all of the following EXCEPT:
    a) putting cells below the surface more rapidly
    b) improving the skin's ability to retain moisture
    c) stimulating blood flow
    d) making the skin smoother _____

13. One should use exfoliation techniques on clients with:
    a) older, thinner skin that can bruise easily
    b) oily skin
    c) skin with many capillaries visible
    d) skin being medically treated _____

14. Enzyme peels differ from AHA treatments in that they:
    a) are harsher and thereby more effective
    b) digest cells both on the surface and below
    c) are more gentle
    d) don't dissolve intercellular glue   _____

15. Which of the following treatments is a combination of an enzyme and a mechanical peeling?
    a) gommage   c) clay mask
    b) powdered enzyme   d) mineral oil   _____

16. Peels are beneficial because they directly help:
    a) cellular functioning
    b) skin with dead cell buildup
    c) fighting bacteria
    d) breaking down glycerine   _____

17. Over-exfoliation CANNOT cause:
    a) inflammation
    b) a breakdown of the body's natural protection
    c) diminished hydration
    d) an increase in cellular functioning   _____

18. What treatment can allow a practitioner to treat several skin conditions at once?
    a) exfoliation   c) mask
    b) emollient   d) antioxidant   _____

19. The hardening component of a mask CANNOT be made of:
    a) alginate   c) papain
    b) gypsum   d) paraffin wax   _____

20. A mask treatment can:
    a) draw impurities from the pores
    b) remove bacteria from the skin
    c) add alcohol to the epidermis
    d) increase blemishes   _____

21. Clay masks are NOT beneficial for:
    a) stimulating circulation   c) antiseptic properties
    b) pore contraction   d) acne inducement   _____

22. The biggest risk when using homemade masks is:
    a) overhydration
    b) an allergic reaction in a client
    c) blemishes
    d) rancid ingredients   _____

23. All of the following can be used to make homemade masks EXCEPT:
    a) eggs   c) preservatives
    b) honey   d) oatmeal   _____

24. One compulsory resource for an esthetician is:
    a) an ingredient dictionary
    b) Internet access
    c) an herb garden
    d) a blood pressure cuff   _____

25. Paraffin masks are beneficial because they:
    a) decrease blood circulation
    b) bring ingredients deeper into the skin
    c) tighten the skin
    d) cool the skin   _____

26. Which ingredients are needed for modelage masks?
    a) gypsum, zinc oxide, water
    b) paraffin, gypsum, water
    c) gypsum, serum, treatment cream
    d) gypsum, treatment cream, water   _____

27. Which of the following is NOT recommended after a modelage mask application?
    a) massage   c) moisturizing treatment
    b) eating   d) hydration   _____

28. Which of the following are NOT included in the makeup of a serum?
    a) vitamins   c) salicyclic acids
    b) lipids   d) antioxidants   _____

29. All of the following are considered moisturizers EXCEPT:
    a) lotions   c) hydrators
    b) elastins   d) creams   _____

30. The types of active ingredients in moisturizers depend on:
    a) the skin type for which they are intended
    b) the type of foundation cream used
    c) the amount of water in the cream
    d) the makeup of the inactive ingredients   _____

31. Water-based moisturizers are ideal for:
    a) skin imbalances   c) biweekly treatments
    b) daily usage   d) diminishing blemishes   _____

32. A valuable ingredient in some day creams is:
    a) mineral oil   c) squalene
    b) papaya   d) sunscreen   _____

33. Night treatment creams generally do NOT have:
    a) a light consistency
    b) additional active ingredients
    c) emollients
    d) a stronger texture   _____

34. What can be blended with massage lotions during treatments?
    a) herbs   c) aromatherapy oils
    b) ampules   d) astringents   _____

35. An ampule extract is applied under:
    a) water   c) a moisturizer
    b) a toner   d) an astringent   _____

36. Sun exposure CANNOT lead to:
    a) collagen production   c) free radical damage
    b) hyperpigmentation   d) elastin deterioration _____

37. An ingredient which helps protect the skin from UVB rays is:
    a) Salicylic acid   c) zinc dioxide
    b) oxybenzone   d) benzyl peroxide   _____

38. Parsol 1789 is an example of:
    a) a preservative   c) an exfolliant
    b) an astringent   d) a sunscreen   _____

39. An SPF of 2 means that a person can stay in the sun how much longer than they normally would?
    a) 4 times as long
    b) 2 hours longer
    c) twice as long
    d) 20% longer
    _____

40. Dihydroxyacetone is an ingredient that reacts with proteins in which type of product?
    a) exfoliating cream
    b) sunscreen
    c) freshener
    d) self-tanning lotion
    _____

41. Which of the following is NOT as important when discussing treatments with a client?
    a) packaging of the products
    b) expectations of the treatment
    c) instructions about the process
    d) precautions before choosing certain treatments
    _____

42. Professional products are often better choices because:
    a) they are easier to find
    b) they have a higher concentration of performance ingredients
    c) they are chosen by professionals
    d) they cost more
    _____

43. A good way to determine product costs is to:
    a) purchase different types of products
    b) consider costs at the end of each year
    c) break them into daily or weekly costs
    d) add product costs up each month
    _____

44. Which of the following should a client NOT use more than two times per week?
    a) exfoliants
    b) cleansers
    c) serums
    d) moisturizers
    _____

45. A good time to pull home-care products for the client would be:
    a) at the beginning of the treatment session
    b) at the one week assessment
    c) while the client is getting dressed
    d) at the post-consultation
    _____

46. When choosing a product line, important factors to consider include all of the following EXCEPT:
    a) pricing
    b) demographics
    c) ingredients
    d) advertising
    _____

47. A preservative is an example of:
    a) an active ingredient
    b) an inactive ingredient
    c) an allergen
    d) an enzyme
    _____

48. All of the following are descriptive terms used in the marketing of skin care EXCEPT:
    a) hypoallergenic
    b) comedogenic
    c) organic
    d) natural
    _____

49. Which ingredients below are more likely to cause a skin reaction?
    a) fragrances
    b) herbs
    c) parabens
    d) paraffins
    _____

50. Which of the following is NOT useful in calming skin reactions?
    a) cold water
    b) cortisone cream
    c) anti-inflammatory products
    d) exfoliants
    _____

51. Colorants can be made up of all of the following ingredients EXCEPT:
    a) vegetable dyes
    b) chemical dyes
    c) pigment dyes
    d) mineral dyes
    _____

52. Which of the following is NOT one of the essential functions of emollients?
    a) prevention of water loss
    b) softening of the skin
    c) filling in the lines of dry skin
    d) instigation of water loss
    _____

53. Which of the following is a humectant used in creams and lotions?
    a) glycerin
    b) methyl paraben
    c) algae
    d) green tea
    _____

54. Which of the following are spreading agents?
    a) humectants
    b) lubricants
    c) fragrances
    d) vehicles
    _____

55. What is the most popular botanical used in cosmetic formulations?
    a) alum
    b) collagen
    c) aloe
    d) lanolin
    _____

56. Benzyl peroxide CANNOT be used:
    a) as a skin allergen
    b) as a hydration agent
    c) to treat blemishes
    d) as an antibacterial agent
    _____

57. A plant extract with calming and soothing properties is:
    a) echinacea
    b) algae
    c) sulfur
    d) chamomile _____

58. Collagen can be derived from which of the following sources?
    a) cow placenta
    b) alcohol
    c) witch hazel
    d) lipids _____

59. Glycerine is formed by a decomposition of:
    a) petroleum hydroxide
    b) hyaluronic acid
    c) oils
    d) propylene glycol _____

60. Which of the following statements about green tea is NOT true?
    a) It is an antioxidant.
    b) It is an antibacterial agent.
    c) It is a stimulant.
    d) It is a depressant. _____

61. Healing, stimulating, soothing, and moisturizing could be the properties of:
    a) licorice
    b) herbs
    c) petroleum jelly
    d) jojoba _____

62. Which ingredient is considered nontoxic, nonsensitizing, and nonirritating?
    a) lavender
    b) rose
    c) tea tree
    d) chamomile _____

63. Which of the following is one of the oldest preservatives in use to combat bacteria and molds?
    a) mineral oil
    b) sodium bicarbonate
    c) methyl paraben
    d) salicylic acid _____

64. Which of the following is NOT one of the forms rose can take?
    a) rose extracts
    b) oil
    c) water
    d) lotions _____

65. Seaweed is NOT known for:
    a) vitamin content
    b) detoxification properties
    c) antifungal properties
    d) moisturizing properties _____

66. Baking soda is also known as:
    a) sodium bicarbonate
    b) sulfur
    c) titanium dioxide
    d) zinc oxide _____

67. What will draw moisture out of the skin if the skin's moisture content is greater than the atmosphere?
    a) silicone
    b) sorbitol
    c) serums
    d) squalane
    _____

68. An ingredient commonly used in acne products is:
    a) titanium dioxide
    b) sodium bicarbonate
    c) witch hazel
    d) sulfur
    _____

69. Titanium dioxide is:
    a) a chemical ingredient that blocks UVB rays
    b) an organic ingredient that darkens skin tone
    c) a nonchemical ingredient that blocks UV rays
    d) a natural ingredient that prevents allergic reactions
    _____

70. Which ingredient is extracted from the bark of the hamanelis shrub?
    a) witch hazel
    b) mint
    c) lavender
    d) eucalyptus
    _____

71. What is a good example of an ingredient that provides a strong barrier against the sun?
    a) potassium hydroxide
    b) zinc oxide
    c) azulene
    d) quaternium 15
    _____

72. Which of the following is NOT a property of plants and herbs?
    a) calming effects
    b) antiseptic effects
    c) exfoliating effects
    d) stimulating effects
    _____

73. When comparing product lines, one should NOT consider:
    a) skin type
    b) quantity
    c) quality of ingredients
    d) texture
    _____

74. Antioxidants are generally applied:
    a) intravenously
    b) orally
    c) surgically
    d) topically
    _____

75. An example of a healing agent would be:
    a) aloe
    b) algae
    c) horse chestnut
    d) mineral oil
    _____

76. Allantoin does NOT:
    a) heal wounds
    b) stimulate tissue growth
    c) lighten pigmentation
    d) treat skin ulcers
    _____

Answer Key

1—d	39—c
2—b	40—d
3—b	41—a
4—d	42—b
5—c	43—c
6—d	44—a
7—a	45—c
8—c	46—d
9—c	47—b
10—c	48—b
11—d	49—a
12—a	50—d
13—b	51—b
14—c	52—d
15—a	53—a
16—b	54—d
17—d	55—c
18—c	56—b
19—c	57—d
20—a	58—a
21—d	59—c
22—b	60—d
23—c	61—b
24—a	62—a
25—b	63—c
26—d	64—d
27—a	65—c
28—c	66—a
29—b	67—b
30—a	68—d
31—b	69—c
32—d	70—a
33—a	71—b
34—c	72—c
35—c	73—b
36—a	74—d
37—b	75—a
38—d	76—c

Chapter 12

THE TREATMENT ROOM

1. Why are the treatment-room checklists important?
   a) State regulations require them to be displayed at all times.
   b) Clients need to know what they are required to do.
   c) Checklists help you remember the many little details involved in setting up, cleaning, and stocking.
   d) There are no such things as treatment-room checklists. _____

2. Because clients form their opinions of you and your business in the first few minutes they see the salon, it is important that you:
   a) Project an air of professionalism: dress neatly and observe good hygiene.
   b) Project an air of popularity: ask your friends to visit.
   c) Hope for the best; you can't affect your clients' opinions in the first few minutes.
   d) The first few minutes are unimportant in forming clients' opinions. _____

3. The most important treatment considerations are:
   a) price, style, and look
   b) state board sanitation regulations and client safety
   c) odor and moisture
   d) every treatment has different considerations _____

4. An esthetician's treatment room chair should be ergonomically correct. This means:
   a) The chair is correct according to state sanitary regulations.
   b) The chair is pleasant to look at and matches the room's décor.
   c) The chair is healthy for the body and spine.
   d) The chair will protect you from macules. _____

5. A dispensary is:
   a) a room for storing and mixing supplies not kept in the treatment room
   b) another word for the treatment room
   c) another word for the esthetician's treatment room chair
   d) an exception to state regulations   _____

6. Facial supplies include:
   a) distilled water, spatulas, and disposable vinyl gloves
   b) seltzer water, comedones, and disposable latex gloves
   c) spring water, scalpels, and reusable vinyl gloves
   d) tap water, whisks, and clear cotton gloves   _____

7. Which of the following items is an optional facial-supply item?
   a) astringent   c) bolster
   b) comedone   d) one pair of eyepads   _____

8. An implement you might use during a facial is:
   a) a comedone implanter   c) a comedone detector
   b) a comedone extractor   d) astringent   _____

9. Which of the following is a disposable facial supply?
   a) comedone extractor   c) cotton gloves
   b) client gown   d) cotton pads   _____

10. A comedone extractor is:
    a) an implement   c) an astringent
    b) a disposable   d) an ergonomic   _____

11. Pads and compresses for facials:
    a) can be made ahead of time and safety stored
    b) must be made at the time of their use
    c) are known as comedones
    d) Pads and compresses are not used in facials.   _____

12. Pads and compresses can be stored overnight:
    a) in open glass bowls
    b) in airtight containers
    c) in your treatment room steamer
    d) Pads and compresses cannot be safely stored overnight.   _____

13. When making cleansing pads:
    a) Cut them so the edges are clean.
    b) Tear them so the edges are frayed.
    c) Make sure they are lumpy, not smooth.
    d) Never make your own cleansing pads.   _____

14. Cotton for eyepads should measure approximately:
    a) 2 inches by 6 inches
    b) 4 inches by 5 inches
    c) 2 inches by 12 inches
    d) There is no standard size for eyepads.   _____

15. Vinyl gloves:
    a) break down in the presence of oils
    b) are ergonomic
    c) are important to have on hand because clients may have
       latex allergies
    d) Vinyl gloves are never used in spas.   _____

16. Basic facial products include:
    a) cleanser, mask, and toner
    b) ergonomic, astringent, and moisturizer
    c) sanitizer and exfoliant
    d) hyperallergenic and sunscreen   _____

17. Equipment preparation in the treatment room includes:
    a) exfoliating   c) emptying the steamer
    b) preheating the steamer   d) turning off the waxer   _____

18. A bolster:
    a) might be something a client wants for arm support
    b) is required for clients' knee support
    c) is used to make facial products stronger
    d) is used to dilute facial products   _____

19. Ergonomics is the study of:
    a) sanitizing equipment
    b) preparing the treatment room
    c) adopting work conditions to suit body and spine health
    d) how different facial products react on the skin   _____

20. Cleansing your hands and placing supplies on the work station is part of:
    a) setting up the treatment room
    b) sanitizing the treatment room
    c) implementing the dispensary
    d) biohazarding   _____

21. Cotton or gauze 4 x 4 pads, sponges, and gloves are:
    a) ergonomics   c) disposables
    b) dispensaries   d) impediments   _____

22. After a facial is over, among the things you should do are:
    a) Conduct the post-consultation and prepare the room
       for the next client.
    b) Have a cup of tea and add up your retail sales commissions.
    c) Place used, soiled disposables in bowls in the dispensary.
    d) Prepare for the next appointment by trying on some of
       the products you'll be using.   _____

23. Equipment sanitation procedures include:
    a) setting out disposables on a clean towel
    b) cleaning all surfaces with a disinfectant
    c) writing up retail sales
    d) putting used disposables in covered waste containers   _____

24. Supply sanitation includes:
    a) sanitizing and refilling the steamer
    b) removing dirty linens and replacing them with clean ones
    c) writing up retail sales
    d) setting supplies out on a clean towel   _____

25. After treatment, implements:
    a) must be put directly in the sanitizer
    b) should be thoroughly washed with an antibacterial soap,
       dried, then put in the sanitizer
    c) should be rinsed and placed back on the appropriate table,
       ready for their next use
    d) must be disposed of in biohazard containers   _____

26. After treatment, soiled gloves and extraction supplies:
    a) should be returned to the dispensary
    b) must be sanitized
    c) must be placed in a sealable plastic bag and then in a covered
       waste container or sharps container
    d) should be placed with the used linens   _____

Answer Key

1—c	15—c
2—a	16—a
3—b	17—b
4—c	18—a
5—a	19—c
6—a	20—a
7—c	21—c
8—b	22—a
9—d	23—a
10—a	24—b
11—a	25—b
12—b	26—c
13—b	
14—a	

Chapter *13*

THE PRINCIPLES OF ESTHETIC PROCEDURES

1. Which statement about massage is true?
   a) You should alternate the number of passes you make for each step.
   b) Classical massage movements are mainly Japanese in tradition.
   c) You should not add movements to your routine once it flows smoothly.
   d) Massage therapists are susceptible to problems because of repetitive movements.   _____

2. Which of the following condition(s) may contraindication a massage?
   a) acne
   b) sunburn
   c) sensitive skin
   d) all of the above are correct   _____

3. What are the five classic massage types?
   a) aromatherapy, reflexology, acupressure, lymph massage, and vibration
   b) effleurage, petrissage, tapotement, Jacquet, and shiatsu
   c) chucking, rolling, wringing, hacking, and slapping
   d) effleurage, petrissage, friction, tapotement, and vibration   _____

4. Which massage is applied with the fingers and palms in a slow and rhythmic manner?
   a) friction
   b) petrissage
   c) tapotement
   d) effleurage   _____

5. Which massage is a generally used on the scalp?
   a) friction
   b) petrissage
   c) tapotement
   d) effleurage   _____

6. Which massage is also known as percussion?
   a) friction
   b) petrissage
   c) tapotement
   d) effleurage   _____

7. Which massage is performed on the more fleshy parts of the face, shoulders, back, and arms?
   a) friction
   b) petrissage
   c) tapotement
   d) effleurage   _____

8. Which type of massage uses essential oils?
   a) tapotement
   b) effleurage
   c) vibration
   d) aromatherapy   _____

9. Which type of massage requires technicians use their bodies and shoulders to create the movement?
   a) shiatsu
   b) effleurage
   c) vibration
   d) acupressure   _____

10. Which type of massage is a rapid shaking movement?
    a) tapotement
    b) effleurage
    c) vibration
    d) aromatherapy   _____

11. Which massage is good for toning sluggish skin?
    a) tapotement
    b) effleurage
    c) vibration
    d) aromatherapy   _____

12. Which massage technique is often used in conjunction with effleurage?
    a) vibration
    b) acupressure
    c) Jacquet
    d) shiatsu   _____

13. Which massage technique is used to treat oily skin?
    a) vibration
    b) acupressure
    c) Jacquet
    d) shiatsu   _____

14. Which massage technique uses the fingers on smaller surfaces and the palms on larger surfaces?
    a) effleurage
    b) petrissage
    c) friction
    d) tapotement   _____

15. Which massage lifts the tissues from their underlying structures, then squeezes, rolls, or pinches them with a light, firm pressure?
    a) effleurage
    b) petrissage
    c) friction
    d) tapotement   _____

16. Which massage uses the techniques of slapping and hacking?
    a) effleurage   c) friction
    b) petrissage   d) tapotement   _____

17. Which massage uses circular movements on the scalp, arms, and hands to stimulate the circulation and glandular activity of the skin?
    a) effleurage   c) friction
    b) petrissage   d) tapotement   _____

18. Friction massage has these variations:
    a) aromatherapy and reflexology movements
    b) checking, rolling, and wringing movements
    c) Jacquet and Shiatsu movements
    d) slapping and hacking movements   _____

19. Which massage is performed for very oily skin?
    a) acupressure   c) Jacquet
    b) Shiatsu   d) lymph   _____

20. Which massage is similar to acupressure and is performed on the hands and feet?
    a) hacking   c) lymph
    b) wringing   d) reflexology   _____

21. Which type of massage helps detoxify the body?
    a) hacking   c) lymph
    b) wringing   d) reflexology   _____

22. What should you do if you need to remove your hands during massage?
    a) apply lotion to them
    b) use aromatherapy
    c) feather them off and on
    d) move them quickly off and on   _____

23. Which statement about massage is NOT true?
    a) an even tempo promotes relaxation
    b) massage from the origin toward the insertion of the muscle
    c) massage toward the heart on the extremities
    d) repeat movements 3-6 times before moving on to the next   _____

24. Which of the following is a pressure point on the face that corresponds to where one movement ends and the next one starts?
    a) the cheeks
    b) the chin
    c) the temples
    d) the eyes   _____

25. Which action is generally performed between steps?
    a) upward and outward strokes on the jawline
    b) circular motions on the chest and neck
    c) applying warm lotion to the face and shoulders
    d) pausing briefly on a pressure point   _____

Answer Key

1—d	14—a
2—d	15—b
3—d	16—d
4—d	17—c
5—a	18—b
6—c	19—c
7—b	20—d
8—d	21—d
9—c	22—c
10—c	23—b
11—a	24—c
12—d	25—d
13—c	

Chapter *14*

BASIC FACIALS AND TREATMENTS

1. What is a core treatment performed by estheticians?
   a) fashion advice
   b) nutrition advice
   c) facials
   d) all of the above are correct _____

2. What are the benefits of a facial?
   a) increased circulation
   b) exfoliation
   c) detoxification
   d) all of the above are correct _____

3. What skill is NOT necessary to give successful facials?
   a) ability to create a nutrition plan
   b) knowledge of skin histology
   c) knowledge of products
   d) ability to analyze skin _____

4. What does the facial treatment protocol include?
   a) makeup consultation
   b) brief client history
   c) explanation of service benefits
   d) stimulating atmosphere _____

5. When you apply facial products, you should:
   a) Work on both sides of the face with moderate pressure, regardless of skin condition.
   b) Work on both sides of the face with the firmest possible touch and pressure.
   c) Concentrate your attention first on the side of the face that needs the least work.
   d) Concentrate your attention first on the side of the face that needs it most. _____

6. What should NOT be part of your relationship with a client?
   a) a professional tone of voice
   b) effort to be friends outside of the workplace
   c) prevention of drips down ears and neck
   d) full attention on client   _____

7. Which personal supplies should clients provide for their facial appointment?
   a) gown   c) lip balm
   b) headband   d) no personal supplies   _____

8. Which products do NOT have to be stocked for facials?
   a) cleanser and toner
   b) makeup and makeup remover
   c) exfoliant and mask
   d) moisturizer and sunscreen   _____

9. What is a good rule for setting up facial supplies?
   a) Set them up differently for each client, according to each client's needs.
   b) They should not be set up; they should be taken off shelves as needed.
   c) They should be set up before the client arrives.
   d) They should be set up as the facial is beginning.   _____

10. When performing a skin analysis, what should you do first?
    a) Look at the skin and observe any obvious conditions.
    b) Touch the skin and note elasticity, softness, etc.
    c) Cleanse the skin.
    d) Choose appropriate products.   _____

11. Contagious diseases are an example of:
    a) an extraction   c) a contraindication
    b) a regiment   d) an inappropriate client   _____

12. What should you drape for the facial?
    a) head   c) hair
    b) chest   d) all of the above are correct   _____

13. Which is the correct order of steps in a facial treatment?
    a) massage, cleanser, toner, warm towels
    b) cleansing, analysis, exfoliation, steam
    c) analysis, cleansing, moisturizer, massage
    d) treatment mask, extractions, exfoliation, analysis   _____

14. How can you make cleansing more effective and enjoyable?
    a) Use warm towels first.
    b) Rub vigorously.
    c) Concentrate on the side with the most-damaged skin.
    d) Allow the client to remain in street clothes.   _____

15. When applying cleansers, how much should you use?
    a) a few drops   c) one tablespoon
    b) one teaspoon   d) one-quarter cup   _____

16. When cleansing, what is the order of application?
    a) begin in center of face, moving to outsides
    b) work down from eyelids to neck
    c) work up from neck to eyelids
    d) begin on outside of face, working in   _____

17. How should cleanser be removed?
    a) with upward strokes
    b) with circular motions
    c) using ten strokes on each cheek
    d) using side-to-side strokes   _____

18. Which area of the face should NOT be subjected to hard pressure?
    a) Adam's apple   c) brow bones
    b) cheekbones   d) nose cartilage   _____

19. When inspecting the skin, what should you look for?
    a) dilated capillaries   c) texture and dryness
    b) evenness of color   d) all of the above are correct   _____

20. What does exfoliation do?
    a) deep-cleanse   c) increase cell turnover rate
    b) extract comedones   d) hydrate skin   _____

21. What helps pores to open?
    a) water   c) papules
    b) warmth   d) clay products   _____

22. Why must papules be removed?
    a) to increase circulation   c) to release bacteria
    b) to soften superficial lines   d) to remove dead cells   _____

23. Which extraction method may NOT be allowed in your state?
    a) lancets
    c) comedone extractors
    b) finger cots
    d) cotton swabs _____

24. How can you achieve optimum success when performing extractions?
    a) Notice which areas of the skin have slanted shafts.
    b) Consistently use the same angle for each pore.
    c) Do not put pressure on skin surrounding the follicular wall.
    d) Do not use comedone extractors. _____

25. What can help soften the plug of cells and debris from the follicular shaft?
    a) cold compress
    c) hydroquinone
    b) sebum solution
    d) enzyme peel _____

26. How many minutes of extractions can most clients tolerate?
    a) 3 to 5
    c) 20 to 30
    b) 10 to 15
    d) 5 to 10 _____

27. When extracting blackheads from the nose, what is important to remember?
    a) Do not be concerned with angles of pores.
    b) Be concerned with only one blackhead at a time.
    c) Press down on cartilage on bridge of nose.
    d) Apply pressure with fingers in a horizontal position. _____

28. Which service increases circulation and metabolism and increases product penetration?
    a) extraction
    c) massage
    b) clay mask
    d) deep cleansing _____

29. What should be used to remove the treatment mask?
    a) cotton compress
    c) toner
    b) steam machine
    d) mushroom electrode _____

30. What should you do before attempting to remove the treatment mask?
    a) Cut the compress vertically from chin to forehead.
    b) Cover the compress with a hot towel.
    c) Massage the compress with an ice cube.
    d) Remove the eyepads. _____

31. Why are serums able to penetrate further into the skin?
    a) Their molecules are smaller.
    b) They are mostly comprised of water.
    c) They are preceded by a vigorous rub to open pores.
    d) They are preceded by a hot towel to open pores.   _____

32. What product can hydrate and balance the skin's oil/water moisture content?
    a) paraffin masks   c) toners
    b) moisturizers   d) sebum   _____

33. Balancing ayurvedic treatments and Chinese face mapping are examples of the philosophy behind which treatment?
    a) acupressure   c) massage
    b) extraction   d) facials   _____

34. When should you perform your sanitation procedures?
    a) the night before
    b) before clients arrive
    c) in the presence of clients
    d) twice daily   _____

35. Using a cotton pad, how should eye makeup be removed?
    a) stroking up and outward
    b) stroking down and outward
    c) stroking down and inward
    d) stroking up and inward   _____

36. After the client's neck and chest have been cleansed, where should you continue?
    a) chin, jaws, cheeks, temples
    b) around nostrils, sides of nose
    c) between brows, across forehead
    d) reapply to neck and chest   _____

37. In what manner should products be applied and removed?
    a) Use both hands on one side, then both hands on the other.
    b) Use both hands at the same time on each side.
    c) Use left hand on left side, then right hand on right side.
    d) Use right hand on left side, then left hand on right side.   _____

38. During the appointment, when is a potential time to exfoliate?
    a) after moisturizing
    b) before initial analysis
    c) after cleansing, before steam
    d) after treatment mask, before toner   _____

39. When should the steamer's ozone be turned on?
    a) before turning on the steamer itself
    b) after steamer is turned on, but before it is steaming
    c) after steamer has begun steaming
    d) does not matter   _____

40. Which type of treatment mask may be appropriate for the eye area?
    a) hydrating   c) stimulating
    b) deep cleansing   d) all of the above are correct   _____

41. If the goal of a client's facial is deep cleansing, what step might you consider omitting?
    a) extractions   c) steam
    b) toner   d) massage   _____

42. What is NOT part of the post-facial checklist?
    a) provide post-consultation c) write up retail sales
    b) wash hands   d) apply client's makeup   _____

43. What can be a quick exfoliating method for a mini-facial?
    a) brush machine   c) thermal mask
    b) hydrating serum   d) disincrustation   _____

44. When treating dry skin, what helps a hydrating serum penetrate?
    a) glycolic peel   c) hydroquinone
    b) galvanic   d) benzoyl peroxide   _____

45. What helps protect the body from free radicals?
    a) lipids   c) antioxidants
    b) water   d) enzyme peel   _____

46. Which ingredient may cause allergies and irritation?
    a) essential oils   c) vitamin C
    b) chamomile   d) licorice extract   _____

47. What calms skin and tones down redness?
    a) lipids
    b) gel mask
    c) brush machine
    d) grapeseed extract
    _____

48. What can improve the appearance of acne-prone skin?
    a) oil-based products and sunscreen
    b) extractions and melanin suppressants
    c) extractions and a good mask
    d) mushroom electrode and demosomes
    _____

49. How does glycolic acid help in acne treatment?
    a) It affects melanin production.
    b) It releases free radical oxygen.
    c) It opens up impaction.
    d) It sterilizes the follicle.
    _____

50. What might you recommend to a client hoping to prevent acne?
    a) Avoid benzoyl peroxide.
    b) Avoid AHAs .
    c) Use more comedogenic products.
    d) Avoid pollution, sun, and humidity.
    _____

51. What can cause hypopigmentation?
    a) overexfoliating
    b) overcleansing
    c) steaming
    d) melanin suppressants
    _____

52. What are the five components of a home-care routine?
    a) cleanse, exfoliate, mask, toner, moisturizer
    b) cleanse, exfoliate, mask, steam, hydroquinone
    c) cleanse, extraction, mask, peel, moisturizer
    d) cleanse, exfoliate, mask, demosomes, moisturizer
    _____

53. How do men's and women's skin-care programs compare?
    a) Men's skin needs less attention.
    b) Men's skin has the same needs.
    c) Men do not need professional skin care.
    d) Men's skin needs more attention.
    _____

54. Men can use toner as they would use which other product?
    a) moisturizer
    b) soap
    c) aftershave
    d) shaving cream
    _____

55. What is true of a man's skin-care regimen?
    a) A man's regimen should begin with only four products.
    b) Tubes are more man-friendly than jars.
    c) Most movements in beard and moustache area should be done against the hair-growth pattern.
    d) Men should shave and wash the face in an upward direction.   _____

56. In what major way do movements for men's treatments differ from movements for women's?
    a) Movements should be downward for men.
    b) Movements should be outward for men.
    c) movements should be from outside in for men.
    d) Direction of movements matters very little for men.   _____

57. What product do men need, but seldom request?
    a) cleansers   c) foamy soaps
    b) eye cream   d) moisturizer   _____

58. What is the treatment goal for folliculitis?
    a) alleviate irritation   c) desensitize the area
    b) disinfect pustules   d) all of the above are correct   _____

59. What are the main areas that men have waxed?
    a) cheeks and brow   c) brow and nape of neck
    b) edge of ears and forehead   d) edge of nose and back   _____

60. What is the best promotion for the esthetics industry?
    a) television advertising   c) product discounts
    b) well-trained technicians   d) treatment discounts   _____

Answer Key

1—c	31—a
2—d	32—b
3—a	33—d
4—c	34—c
5—a	35—b
6—b	36—a
7—d	37—b
8—b	38—c
9—c	39—c
10—a	40—a
11—c	41—d
12—d	42—d
13—b	43—a
14—a	44—b
15—b	45—c
16—c	46—a
17—a	47—b
18—d	48—c
19—d	49—c
20—c	50—d
21—b	51—a
22—c	52—a
23—a	53—b
24—a	54—c
25—d	55—b
26—b	56—a
27—b	57—b
28—c	58—d
29—a	59—c
30—c	60—b

Chapter 15

MACHINES

1. A magnifying lamp is also known as a:
   a) Wood's lamp
   b) skin scope
   c) diopter
   d) loupe   _____

2. The magnification power of a loupe is measured in:
   a) amperes
   b) watts
   c) diopters
   d) volts   _____

3. What is the most commonly used diopter lamp?
   a) 3-diopter
   b) 5-diopter
   c) 10-diopter
   d) 20-diopter   _____

4. What is a Wood's lamp used for?
   a) to treat oily skin conditions
   b) to warm the skin during a facial massage
   c) to tone dry, wrinkled skin
   d) to illuminate skin conditions that are usually invisible   _____

5. The main purpose of the rotary brush is to:
   a) deeply cleanse clogged pores
   b) stimulate muscle contractions
   c) lightly exfoliate the skin
   d) remove surface facial hair   _____

6. In addition to cleansing impurities, the vacuum machine:
   a) helps to reduce creases and laugh lines
   b) softens the skin
   c) closes the pores
   d) oxygenates the skin   _____

7. Spray mists:
   a) enhance product penetration
   b) stimulate muscle contractions
   c) calm and hydrate the skin
   d) sanitize the skin   _____

8. To have an antiseptic effect, steamers must contain:
   a) ozone   c) minerals
   b) distilled water   d) freshener solution   _____

9. What does ozone consist of?
   a) one oxygen atom   c) three oxygen atoms
   b) two oxygen atoms   d) four oxygen atoms   _____

10. The usual treatment time for a steamer is:
    a) 2 to 5 minutes   c) 12 to 15 minutes
    b) 6 to 10 minutes   d) about 20 minutes   _____

11. What is the correct way to use essential oils with a steamer?
    a) adding them directly to the water
    b) adding a few drops to the mouth of the nozzle
    c) putting a few drops on the client's skin
    d) placing the oil in a separate container away from the steamer   _____

12. Neglected steamers have a tendency to spit hot water because of the:
    a) use of distilled water
    b) use of tap water
    c) buildup of mineral deposits
    d) tendency for the heating element to overheat   _____

13. Mineral deposits may appear as a:
    a) white or yellow crusty film on the heating element
    b) collection of black spots at the mouth of the nozzle
    c) green, moldy coating on the steamer jar
    d) thick, rusty-colored streak on the heating element   _____

14. A Lucas sprayer produces a mist that is:
    a) cool   c) fine
    b) antiseptic   d) heavy   _____

15. The frequency of a high-frequency current is measured in:
    a) joules   c) watts
    b) ampoules   d) hertz   _____

16. A high-frequency process for permanent hair removal is:
    a) anaphoresis   c) cataphoresis
    b) thermolysis   d) iontophoresis   _____

17. A high-frequency apparatus:
    a) stimulates circulation   c) hydrates dry skin
    b) stimulates motor nerves   d) cools the skin   _____

18. The tube of a high-frequency electrode contains:
    a) mostly air   c) mostly argon gas
    b) an air vacuum   d) mostly neon gas   _____

19. The best way to clean a glass electrode is by:
    a) immersing it directly in soapy water
    b) placing it in an ultraviolet machine
    c) wiping it with a solution of soap and water
    d) placing it in an autoclave   _____

20. The galvanic machine converts current from an electrical outlet
    to one that:
    a) oscillates rapidly
    b) flows continuously in one direction
    c) alternates asymetrically
    d) has no polarity   _____

21. What is the term for a galvanic process that emulsifies sebum
    and debris?
    a) saponification   c) thermolysis
    b) iontophoresis   d) disincrustation   _____

22. What is saponification?
    a) a specialized process for deep pore cleansing
    b) a method of treatment for skin with pustular acne
    c) a chemical reaction that transforms sebum into soap
    d) a relatively new process for hydrating dry, wrinkled skin   _____

23. The ionizing roller is a popular:
    a) pressurized wand   c) disincrustator
    b) laser tool   d) electrode   _____

24. What area of the face should be avoided during iontophoresis?
    a) the cheeks   c) the chin area
    b) the T-zone   d) the forehead   _____

25. The separation of a substance into positive and negative ions
    is called:
    a) magnetic response   c) iontophoresis
    b) thermolysis   d) ionization   _____

26. Products with an alkaline tendency are:
    a) neutral   c) positive
    b) negative   d) alternating   _____

27. Permeability refers to the:
    a) quality of skin tone
    b) molecular weight of a product
    c) ability of a product to penetrate skin
    d) solubility of a product   _____

28. The infusion of a negative product into the skin is known as:
    a) anaphoresis   c) iontophoresis
    b) cataphoresis   d) thermolysis   _____

29. To ensure proper electrical connections during iontophoresis, it is
    important to:
    a) place a metallic electrode directly on the skin
    b) moisten electrodes with gauze or a sponge
    c) have the client and the esthetician hold electrodes
       with the same charge
    d) turn on the current before handing the electrode to the client _____

30. When using the ionto mask, a wet pad is placed:
    a) on the client's forehead
    b) under the client's shoulder
    c) on the back of the client's hand
    d) on the client's inner arm   _____

31. The heat mask provides:
    a) a gentle surface massage
    b) an antiseptic effect on the skin
    c) a soothing heat to hydrate the skin
    d) a relaxing heat that penetrates deeply   _____

32. Microcurrent machines are helpful in treating such conditions as:
    a) psoriasis
    b) Bell's Palsy
    c) impetigo
    d) pustular acne _____

33. What treatment is popular with women who want a glowing complexion for special events?
    a) paraffin wax
    b) ionto mask
    c) heat mask
    d) light therapy _____

34. Towel cabinets should be cleaned with:
    a) white vinegar and distilled water
    b) white vinegar and baking soda
    c) topical disinfectant or 70% alcohol spray
    d) plain soap and water _____

35. An add-on service that complements salon treatments is:
    a) a paraffin wax
    b) a heat mask
    c) the Lucas spray
    d) heated boots and mitts _____

36. A powerful electronic vacuum that sprays high-grade crystals across the skin's surface with a pressurized wand is:
    a) the microdermabrasion machine
    b) the vaccum spray
    c) the Lucas sprayer
    d) wave therapy _____

37. Improper use of microdermabrasion can cause:
    a) dry, flaky skin
    b) coarse textured skin
    c) facial lines and wrinkles
    d) hyperpigmentation _____

38. Lasers:
    a) have mostly topical uses
    b) have a gentle overall effect on the skin
    c) work precisely in a given area
    d) create a chemical reaction _____

39. In light therapy, red lights are considered:
    a) stimulating
    b) calming
    c) irritating
    d) cooling _____

40. Steamers should be cleaned:
    a) every day
    b) once a week
    c) once a month
    d) bimonthly _____

Answer Key

1—d	21—d
2—c	22—c
3—b	23—d
4—d	24—a
5—c	25—d
6—a	26—b
7—c	27—c
8—a	28—a
9—c	29—b
10—b	30—b
11—b	31—c
12—c	32—b
13—a	33—a
14—c	34—c
15—d	35—b
16—b	36—a
17—a	37—d
18—d	38—c
19—c	39—a
20—b	40—d

Chapter *16*

HAIR REMOVAL

1. Which of the following is NOT true about cosmetic hair removal?
   a) It has been practiced since ancient times.
   b) It was first performed in Egypt.
   c) Generally only women experience unwanted hair growth.
   d) It can be as much as 50% of a salon's business.   _____

2. To increase race times, male swimmers might have hair removed from their:
   a) bikini lines   c) face
   b) legs   d) naval   _____

3. Which of the following should be your primary concern when choosing a hair removal method?
   a) the latest trend
   b) a client's previous experience
   c) ease of completion
   d) health and safety   _____

4. The scientific study of hair is:
   a) papillology   c) pilology
   b) trichology   d) vellusology   _____

5. Which of the following is NOT a part of the hair structure?
   a) lanugo   c) follicle
   b) arrector pili muscle   d) bulb   _____

6. Which of the following is NOT true about all follicles?
   a) They are shaped as small tubes.
   b) They are made up of epidermal cells.
   c) They contain hair shafts.
   d) They are slanted.   _____

7. The lower part of the hair root is the:
   a) papilla   c) muscle
   b) blood vessel   d) bulb   _____

8. Which of the following is NOT needed for hair growth?
   a) light   c) minerals
   b) nutrients   d) vitamins   _____

9. A face contains how many follicles per square inch?
   a) 32   c) 3200
   b) 320   d) 32,000   _____

10. Although the term "lanugo" means the hair that grows on a
    fetus before birth, it is sometimes also used to describe:
    a) coarse dark hair   c) facial hair
    b) fine downy hair   d) newly growing hair   _____

11. Which of the following is a stage of hair growth?
    a) anagen   c) telogen
    b) catagen   d) all of the above are correct   _____

12. Which of the following is true about the telogen stage of hair growth?
    a) hair falls out   c) hair is limp in its follicle
    b) hair is active   d) hair is still growing   _____

13. For what length of time does hair grow before it reaches the
    surface of the skin?
    a) 4-13 hours   c) 4-13 weeks
    b) 4-13 days   d) 4-13 months   _____

14. If a client wants to have his or her hair cut each time it grows out
    an inch, it is likely that he or she will have a cut:
    a) every two weeks   c) every six weeks
    b) once a month   d) every two months   _____

15. If a client asks why his or her hair is lifeless and dull, you might gently
remind the client that this might be a sign of:
   a) overexposure to heat
   c) overexposure to cold
   b) ill health
   d) aging _____

16. A female client who has moderate hirsutism could:
   a) be pregnant
   b) be vitamin deficient
   c) be suffering from a hormone imbalance
   d) all of the above are correct _____

17. Because the body needs the kind of hair that can protect it from
the intensity of the ultraviolet rays with which it is faced:
   a) people in Ireland and Sweden tend to have coarse hair
   b) people who live near the equator tend to have fine hair
   c) people in Africa and Australia tend to have dark coarse hair
   d) central Europeans often have light colored hair _____

18. Graying hair:
   a) is harder to remove than before it turned gray because
   the root system increases by 50%
   b) is easier to remove than before it turned gray because
   the root system decreases by 50%
   c) is harder to remove than before it turned gray because
   there is more of it
   d) is easier to remove than before it turned gray because
   there is less of it _____

19. Permanent hair removal is generally done:
   a) at home
   c) in a salon
   b) in a medical setting
   d) in a hospital _____

20. If a client wishes to have hair removal be truly permanent what
should you recommend?
   a) electrolysis
   c) photo light
   b) laser
   d) pulsed light _____

21. How does the Galvanic method of electrolysis work?
    a) An electrical charge burns the follicle and allows easy hair removal.
    b) An electrical charge transforms saline in the follicle into sodium chloride, which weakens the hold of the follicle wall and allows easy hair removal.
    c) A high-frequency current produces heat, which coagulates and destroys the hair follicle.
    d) High frequency and direct current are sent together through a fine needle or probe to destroy the hair follicle. _____

22. To perform electrolysis you will need:
    a) standard esthetician training
    b) special training
    c) standard esthetician training and licensing
    d) special training and licensing _____

23. When is laser hair removal most effective?
    a) when hair is in the anagen stage
    b) when hair is in the catagen stage
    c) when hair is in the telogen stage
    d) when hair is in the lanugo stage _____

24. Since they remove hair by breaking the contact between the bulb and the papilla, tweezing, waxing, and sugaring are all methods of:
    a) epilation   c) thermolysis
    b) depilation   d) vellusation _____

25. Which of the following is NOT true about shaving?
    a) It can be a skin irritant.
    b) It can cause ingrown hairs.
    c) It causes hair to grow back more thickly.
    d) It removes hair only at the skin's surface. _____

26. How would you suggest a client solve an ongoing Barbae folliculitis problem?
    a) He should use a different shaving tool.
    b) He should use a different shaving cream.
    c) He should shave less often.
    d) He should shave in a different direction. _____

27. Which method of hair removal uses a caustic alkali solution?
    a) electrolysis   c) depilation
    b) epilation   d) thermolysis _____

28. Depilatory creams and lotions are generally used:
    a) in a medical setting
    b) in clients' homes
    c) in a hospital
    d) in a salon   _____

29. In what direction should the hair be pulled when tweezing?
    a) at an angle in the direction in which it is growing
    b) at an angle in the opposite direction from which it is growing
    c) straight out from the skin
    d) none of the above are correct   _____

30. To ensure that the hair has been completely removed when tweezing, it's important to check your work with:
    a) a gloved finger
    b) an ungloved finger
    c) a magnifying glass
    d) a magnifying light   _____

31. Which of the following is the correct way to apply and remove hard or soft wax?
    a) Apply the wax in the direction in which the hair is growing and peel the wax in the direction in which you applied it.
    b) Apply the wax in the opposite direction from which the hair is growing and peel the wax in the direction in which you applied it.
    c) Apply the wax in the direction in which the hair is growing and peel the wax in the opposite direction.
    d) Apply the wax in the opposite direction from which the hair is growing and peel the wax in the direction in which the hair is growing.   _____

32. If a resin-based wax you are applying to a client's upper lip accidentally splashes onto lanugo hair on the cheek near the hairline, how will you remove it?
    a) Allow the wax to harden and then scrape it off gently so the hair remains.
    b) Dissolve the wax with oil and then wipe it away.
    c) Allow the wax to reach a soft stage and then pull it off quickly so the hair remains.
    d) Allow the wax to harden and remove it and the lanugo hair as usual.   _____

33. Hard waxes are NOT available as:
    a) pellets
    b) sticks
    c) strips
    d) blocks   _____

34. Which of the following is NOT used for wax removal?
    a) linen
    b) cotton
    c) pellon
    d) muslin   _____

35. When removing hair for a client using the warm waxing method, how long will you wait after you apply the wax to remove the strips?
    a) The strips should be removed immediately.
    b) The strips should be removed after they've cooled for five minutes.
    c) The strips should be removed after they've cooled for ten minutes.
    d) The strips should be removed after they've completely hardened. _____

36. Many estheticians prefer a roll-on waxer because it is:
    a) less messy and less expensive
    b) more sanitary and faster
    c) less messy and more sanitary
    d) less expensive and faster _____

37. Sugaring is still a popular method of hair removal because it:
    a) works well for those with sensitive skin
    b) is water soluble
    c) is more comfortable than wax because it adheres to the hair only
    d) all of the above are correct _____

38. Why would a client's skin blister during waxing?
    a) The client is allergic.
    b) The client's hair is too coarse to pull away from the follicle without tugging.
    c) The wax is too hot.
    d) The wax is not removed soon enough. _____

39. Before you begin a waxing treatment, it is important that you:
    a) have your client sign a waiver
    b) do a patch test on the client's skin
    c) put on disposable gloves
    d) all of the above are correct _____

40. A step-stool is useful when waxing legs because it allows:
    a) the client to raise one leg at a time
    b) the esthetician to lean easily over both legs
    c) the client to get on and off the table easily
    d) the esthetician to reach supplies as needed _____

41. Pointed tip tweezers are the best instrument for:
    a) shaping eyebrows
    b) removing ingrown hairs
    c) removing hair from upper lips
    d) removing hair from a bikini line   _____

42. Why are stainless steel tweezers the best choice for a discerning salon?
    a) The points on stainless steel tweezers stay sharp.
    b) Stainless steel tweezers retain their flexibility.
    c) Stainless steel tweezers won't corrode in an autoclave.
    d) Stainless steel tweezers can be cleaned with household bleach. _____

43. At a minimum, after each use, tweezers must be:
    a) immersed in hospital-strength disinfectant
    b) immersed in household-strength disinfectant
    c) wiped with hospital-strength disinfectant
    d) wiped with household-strength disinfectant   _____

44. Which method of hair removal relies on radio waves?
    a) electrolysis   c) thermolysis
    b) electronic tweezers   d) none of the above
                                          are correct   _____

45. If you find that the wax removal strips you are using shed or
    stretch too much, you might consider switching to:
    a) pellon   c) muslin
    b) cotton   d) linen   _____

46. What is the purpose of pre-waxing preparation solutions?
    a) to desensitize the skin   c) to soothe the skin
    b) to calm the client   d) to sanitize the skin   _____

47. When should a hair growth inhibitor be applied?
    a) in the salon before waxing
    b) in the salon after waxing
    c) in the salon during waxing
    d) after the client returns home   _____

48. If forceful pulling on a hair that is being removed causes blood or fluid to appear on the surface of the client's skin, which of the following must you do?
    a) Stop the bleeding with tea tree antiseptic or other styptic.
    b) Sterilize non-disposable implements.
    c) Dispose of disposable implements in a hazardous waste container.
    d) all of the above are correct   _____

49. A client with varicose veins:
    a) should not have his or her legs waxed
    b) should not use chemical depilatories
    c) should wax rather than shave his or her legs
    d) should not remove hair from his or her legs   _____

50. A client who has a history of cold sores:
    a) should use chemical hair removal treatments only
    b) should not have facial waxing
    c) should not shave facial hair
    d) should not have waxing on any areas of the body   _____

51. Before you treat a client it is important that you know whether he or she:
    a) uses any topical medications
    b) uses any oral medication
    c) has any allergies or sensitivities
    d) all of the above are correct   _____

52. How often should you ask a client about their medical history?
    a) annually   c) at each visit
    b) twice a year   d) during the first visit   _____

53. How long should hair be to be effectively removed by waxing?
    a) under 1/4"
    b) between 1/4" and 1/2"
    c) over 1/2"
    d) the length of the hair to be removed doesn't matter   _____

54. How thickly should hard wax be applied?
    a) about as thick as a dime with a thinner end for pulling
    b) about as thick as a dime with a thicker end for pulling
    c) about as thick as a nickel with a thinner end for pulling
    d) about as thick as a nickel with a thicker end for pulling   _____

55. If a patient seems very uncomfortable during wax removal, try:
    a) holding the skin tighter   c) lifting up while pulling
    b) pulling more slowly   d) using cooler wax   _____

56. How often should the thermostat on a wax heater be checked?
    a) annually   c) after every five uses
    b) monthly   d) before each use   _____

57. If a client wants to keep his or her eyebrows neatly tweezed
    you should suggest:
    a) that he or she schedules a weekly appointment
    b) that he or she tweezes stray hairs at home on a daily basis
    c) that he or she schedules a biweekly appointment
    d) that he or she schedules a monthly appointment and
       tweezes stray hairs on a weekly basis   _____

58. Which of the following is a good product for helping wax adhere
    to hair?
    a) talcum powder   c) cornstarch
    b) emollient cream   d) tea tree oil   _____

59. Underarm waxing is different from waxing other body parts because:
    a) the skin is more sensitive
    b) the hair is more coarse
    c) the hair grows in different directions
    d) sweat makes it hard for wax to adhere   _____

60. It's important to avoid waxing over moles because:
    a) A hair growing from a mole is too coarse to be removed.
    b) Moles are highly sensitive, and the client will feel pain.
    c) Moles bleed easily and you risk spreading contagions.
    d) The mole can be traumatized and cause future problems
       for the client.   _____

Answer Key

1—c	31—c
2—b	32—b
3—d	33—c
4—b	34—a
5—a	35—a
6—c	36—c
7—d	37—d
8—a	38—c
9—c	39—d
10—b	40—c
11—d	41—b
12—a	42—c
13—c	43—a
14—d	44—b
15—b	45—a
16—d	46—d
17—c	47—b
18—a	48—d
19—b	49—a
20—a	50—b
21—b	51—d
22—d	52—c
23—a	53—b
24—a	54—d
25—c	55—a
26—d	56—b
27—c	57—a
28—b	58—c
29—a	59—c
30—d	60—d

Chapter *17*

ADVANCED ESTHETICS TOPICS: AN INDUSTRY OVERVIEW

1. What leads to premature aging?
   - a) antioxidants
   - b) free radicals
   - c) dimethylaminoethanol
   - d) alpha lipoic acid _____

2. What best describes free radicals?
   - a) vitamins, amino acids, and other natural substances
   - b) stimulate fibroblasts, cells that produce collagen and elastin
   - c) increase chemicals that control muscle tone, which improves the appearance of sagging skin
   - d) aggressive, unstable, oxygen-containing molecules _____

3. What best describes DMAE?
   - a) vitamins, amino acids, and other natural substances
   - b) stimulates fibroblasts, cells that produce collagen and elastin
   - c) boosts the effects of other antioxidants
   - d) aggressive, unstable, oxygen-containing molecules _____

4. What best describes vitamin C ester?
   - a) vitamins, amino acids, and other natural substances
   - b) stimulates fibroblasts, cells that produce collagen and elastin
   - c) boosts the effects of other antioxidants
   - d) aggressive, unstable, oxygen-containing molecules _____

5. Which antioxidant strengthens the white blood cells?
   - a) DMAE
   - b) vitamin C (L- ascorbic acid)
   - c) vitamin C ester
   - d) alpha lipoic acid _____

6. Which antioxidant increases chemicals that control muscle tone, which improves the appearance of sagging skin?
   - a) DMAE
   - b) vitamin C (L- ascorbic acid)
   - c) vitamin C Ester
   - d) alpha lipoic acid _____

7. Which antioxidant is also anti-inflammatory, which reduces redness?
   a) DMAE
   b) vitamin C (L- ascorbic acid)
   c) vitamin C ester
   d) alpha lipoic acid   _____

8. Which is NOT a procedure used by Skin Care Therapists (Estheticians)?
   a) superficial peeling   c) deep peels
   b) exfoliation   d) keratolysis   _____

9. What is the Cell Renewal Factor (CRF) for people over 50?
   a) 84-126 days   c) 21-28 days
   b) 28-42 days   d) 42-84 days   _____

10. Which type of exfoliation is mainly used on scars?
    a) Jessner's   c) phenol
    b) dermabrasion   d) TCA   _____

11. Which type of exfoliation is a superficial peel?
    a) Jessner's   c) phenol
    b) dermabrasion   d) TCA   _____

12. Which type of exfoliation is a medium depth peel?
    a) Jessner's   c) phenol
    b) dermabrasion   d) TCA   _____

13. Which type of exfoliation is a highly acidic deep peel?
    a) Jessner's   c) phenol
    b) dermabrasion   d) TCA   _____

14. What is the average pH of normal skin?
    a) 5.5   c) 7
    b) 6   d) ranges from 8-14   _____

15. Which matter is NOT found in intercellular cement?
    a) lipids   c) glycoproteins
    b) malic acid   d) active enzymes   _____

16. Which statement is NOT true about peels?
    a) They improve the texture of the skin.
    b) They control skin conditions such as acne.
    c) They help heal sunburn.
    d) They reduce fine lines.   _____

17. What ingredients might you combine with peels for mature and/or sensitive skin?
    a) glycolic acid, lactic acid, salicylic acid, azelaic acid
    b) bearberry extract, azelaic acid, ascorbic acid
    c) phosopholipids, linoleic acid, aloe vera, allantoin, kojic acid, licorice root
    d) glycolic acid, hydroquinone 2%, kojic acid, licorice root, mulberry extract   _____

18. What ingredients might you combine with peels for acne?
    a) glycolic acid, lactic acid, salicylic acid, azelaic acid
    b) glycolic acid, lactic acid, ceramides, hyaluronic acid
    c) phosopholipids, linoleic acid, aloe vera, allantoin, kojic acid, licorice root
    d) glycolic acid, hydroquinone 2%, kojic acid, licorice root, mulberry extract   _____

19. What is a true statement about peels?
    a) They hydrate the skin.
    b) It can take approximately 3 months to notice a difference in the skin.
    c) More than 12 weekly peels in a row is not recommended.
    d) Peels are typically not recommended during the hot months.   _____

20. Which peel is best for ultra-sensitive skin?
    a) glycolic acid   c) tartaric acid
    b) enzyme   d) benzoyl peroxide   _____

21. What is the hormone that is key to the good health and appearance of female skin?
    a) botox   c) estrogen
    b) collagen   d) endermology   _____

22. Estrogen from plants is called:
    a) desmosomes   c) phytoestrogens
    b) hydrotherapy   d) endermology   _____

23. Which is NOT a plant source of estrogen?
    a) butcher's broom   c) Mexican wild yam
    b) licorice root   d) lavender root   _____

24. Which ingredient is NOT known to have a positive effect on mature and rosacea skin?
    a) green tea   c) mud
    b) seaweed   d) chamomile   _____

25. Which treatment uses ancient Indian concepts and ingredients suited to the three body/mind types?
    a) balneotherapy
    b) hydrotherapy
    c) aromatherapy
    d) ayurvedic _____

26. Which treatment uses water in its three forms, (ice, steam and liquid) either internally or externally?
    a) balneotherapy
    b) hydrotherapy
    c) aromatherapy
    d) ayurvedic _____

27. Which treatment uses mud or fango, Dead Sea salt, seeweed, enzymes, or peat baths?
    a) balneotherapy
    b) hydrotherapy
    c) aromatherapy
    d) ayurvedic _____

28. Which statement best describes Botox treatment?
    a) a neuromuscular treatment often used on frown lines between the eyes
    b) a treatment for cellulite that can be given before and after liposuction
    c) usually a bovine derivative used to fill in wrinkles or to make lips larger
    d) wrinkle treatments using intense pulsed light _____

29. Which statement best describes nonablative treatment?
    a) a neuromuscular treatment often used on frown lines between the eyes
    b) a treatment for cellulite that can be given before and after liposuction
    c) usually a bovine derivative used to fill in wrinkles or to make lips larger
    d) wrinkle treatments using intense pulsed light _____

30. Which statement best describes endermology treatment?
    a) a neuromuscular treatment often used on frown lines between the eyes
    b) a treatment for cellulite that can be given before and after liposuction
    c) usually a bovine derivative used to fill in wrinkles or to make lips larger
    d) wrinkle treatments using intense pulsed light _____

Answer Key

1—b	16—c
2—d	17—c
3—c	18—a
4—b	19—d
5—b	20—b
6—a	21—c
7—d	22—c
8—c	23—d
9—d	24—c
10—b	25—d
11—a	26—b
12—d	27—a
13—c	28—a
14—a	29—d
15—b	30—b

Chapter *18*

THE WORLD OF MAKEUP

1. When designing a makeup "look" for a client, some things you'll
   need to take into account include:
   a) the client's lifestyle
   b) the client's food preferences
   c) your preferences
   d) how good a customer the client is   _____

2. Opportunities in the field of makeup include work in:
   a) film   c) ergonomics
   b) photosynthesis   d) botany   _____

3. High-quality makeup:
   a) is otherwise known as camouflage makeup
   b) is only used on photo shoots
   c) glides on easily
   d) is the least expensive kind   _____

4. Foundation protects the skin from:
   a) skin eruptions from acne or allergies
   b) food impurities and allergies
   c) climate, dirt, and pollution
   d) foundation does not protect the skin   _____

5. For normal-to-dry skin:
   a) oil-based foundation is recommended
   b) oil-free foundation is recommended
   c) no foundation should be used
   d) no foundation can be used   _____

6. Cream foundations are:
   a) generally suited for dry-to-normal skin
   b) generally suited for oily-to-dry skin
   c) generally suited for oily skin
   d) generally suited for all skin types   _____

7. Skin tones are classified as:
   a) cold, medium, and hot   c) cool, neutral, and warm
   b) light, average, and heavy   d) pale, medium, and tan   _____

8. Foundations should:
   a) always be chosen as closely as possible to the opposite of the skin tone
   b) always be chosen as closely as possible to the actual skin tone
   c) always be chosen 2–3 shades darker than the actual skin tone
   d) be chosen in any shade the client prefers   _____

9. Pot concealer:
   a) gives sheer-to-medium coverage
   b) gives light-to-warm coverage
   c) is the lightest type of concealer
   d) is the heaviest and provides the most coverage   _____

10. Concealers:
    a) control acne outbreaks   c) cover blemishes
    b) bleach discolorations   d) conceal under-eye bags   _____

11. Face powder:
    a) adds a glossy finish to the face
    b) adds a dull finish to the face
    c) disappears onto the skin
    d) bleaches discolorations   _____

12. For dry-to-normal skin:
    a) Light and medium weight powders are generally best.
    b) Heavy and medium weight powders are generally best.
    c) Oil-free powders are best.
    d) No special powder is recommended.   _____

13. Cream or gel cheek colors:
    a) impart a matte finish
    b) are the most widely used
    c) are generally recommended for dry and normal skin
    d) are oil-free   _____

14. Stick and cream eye shadows contain:
    a) litmus
    b) macules
    c) petrolatum
    d) humectants _____

15. Darker shades of eye shadow:
    a) create a flat field of color
    b) make the iris appear lighter
    c) make the iris appear darker
    d) are oil-heavy _____

16. A highlight eye shadow is:
    a) lighter than the client's skin tone
    b) darker than the client's skin tone
    c) close to the client's skin tone
    d) oil-free _____

17. Eyeliner is used to:
    a) make the eyes appear lighter
    b) make the eyes appear glossier
    c) make the eyes appear larger
    d) make the eyes appear smaller _____

18. When preparing an eyeliner or eyebrow pencil for use:
    a) Wipe the pencil with a clean tissue, sharpen it, and sanitize the sharpener.
    b) Sharpen the pencil, wipe it with a clean tissue, and dispose of the sharpener.
    c) Sanitize the sharpener, sharpen the pencil, and wipe with a clean tissue.
    d) Wipe with a clean tissue and sharpen if needed. _____

19. The best color choice for eyebrow pencils is usually:
    a) gold
    b) brown
    c) black
    d) silver _____

20. Mascara is available in:
    a) liquid, dry, and pressed powder
    b) liquid, gel, and cream
    c) liquid, cake, and cream
    d) liquid, pencil, and powder _____

21. When applying mascara:
    a) Use a sanitized, reusable wand.
    b) Use an eyelash curler.
    c) Use a disposable wand.
    d) Use a clean tissue. _____

22. The primary ingredient in lipsticks is:
    a) carnauba wax   c) castor oil
    b) petroleum   d) lecithin   _____

23. To keep lip color from feathering:
    a) Use a heavy concealer.   c) Use a lipliner.
    b) Use a heavy foundation.   d) Use a lipstick concealer.   _____

24. Most eye makeups are:
    a) water-based   c) oil-resistant
    b) water-resistant   d) wax-based   _____

25. Greasepaint and pancake makeup are:
    a) heavy   c) water-based
    b) light   d) loose powders   _____

26. Makeup brushes are made of:
    a) synthetic or animal fibers
    b) cotton and wool fibers
    c) plant fibers
    d) oil-based and water-based fibers   _____

27. A brush that is narrow and firm with a flat edge is a:
    a) lash brush   c) concealer brush
    b) brow brush   d) powder brush   _____

28. To clean makeup brushes:
    a) Keep the ferrule pointing down.
    b) Keep the ferrule pointing up.
    c) Keep the ferrule pointing horizontal.
    d) Remove the ferrule.   _____

29. Among the colors that color wheels show are:
    a) elementary colors
    b) complementary colors
    c) neutral colors
    d) contractual colors   _____

30. A pair of primary and secondary colors directly opposite each
    other on the color wheel are called:
    a) contrasting   c) tertiary
    b) neutral   d) complementary   _____

31. Colors with a yellow undertone are:
    a) neutral
    b) complementary
    c) warm
    d) cool
    _____

32. Reds and greens are:
    a) warm colors
    b) cool colors
    c) tertiary colors
    d) both warm and cool
    _____

33. Skin color may be:
    a) pale, medium, or tan
    b) light, medium, or dark
    c) light, neutral, or bright
    d) neutral or complementary
    _____

34. To create a soft, natural look, if skin color is light, use:
    a) light colors
    b) medium colors
    c) complementary colors
    d) blue colors
    _____

35. The safest choices in recommending colors are:
    a) light tones
    b) warm tones
    c) cool tones
    d) neutral tones
    _____

36. Complementary colors for blue eyes contain:
    a) blues and greens
    b) yellows and reds
    c) neutrals
    d) violets
    _____

37. If you have chosen cool colors for eye makeup, cheek and lip colors should be:
    a) cool
    b) warm
    c) major
    d) minor
    _____

38. The artistically ideal face is:
    a) round
    b) oval
    c) pear-shaped
    d) square
    _____

39. A wide forehead and a narrow, pointed chin characterize a face that is:
    a) round
    b) oval
    c) inverted triangle
    d) square
    _____

40. When applying corrective makeup, to accent a feature:
    a) Use a concealer or pencil that is lighter than the foundation.
    b) Use a concealer or pencil that is darker than the foundation.
    c) Use a concealer or pencil that is the same tone as the foundation.
    d) Use no makeup in addition to the foundation.
    _____

41. To avoid makeup transfer onto the client's clothes, always set with:
    a) an oil-based cream
    b) a water-based foundation
    c) a translucent powder
    d) a neutral gel _____

42. To correct a broad jawline:
    a) Apply a darker shade of foundation over the heavy area of the jaw.
    b) Apply a lighter shade of foundation over the heavy area of the jaw.
    c) Use a darker foundation on the neck.
    d) Use a darker foundation on the sides of the nose. _____

43. The ideal eyebrow shape can be determined by:
    a) 2 lines
    b) 3 lines
    c) 4 lines
    d) the client's preference _____

44. Extending eyebrows outward:
    a) makes eyes appear closer together
    b) makes eyes appear farther apart
    c) makes eyes appear smaller
    d) makes eyes appear larger _____

45. Ruddy skin:
    a) is skin with a red tone
    b) is skin with a blue tone
    c) is skin with a yellow tone
    d) is skin with a green tone _____

46. The client consultation:
    a) is the first step in the makeup process
    b) is the last step in the makeup process
    c) may be conducted while you apply the client's makeup
    d) may be conducted at any point in the appointment _____

47. Natural light is the:
    a) most difficult to apply makeup in
    b) best light to apply makeup in
    c) worst light to apply makeup in
    d) The source of light does not matter. _____

48. When applying powder, blush, and eye shadow, you can get better control and blending with:
    a) sponges
    b) fingertips
    c) brushes
    d) cotton swabs _____

49. When removing products like concealer or lipstick from jars or containers:
    a) Dispose of the container after you've used it on the client.
    b) Use a brush.
    c) Use a clean spatula.
    d) Ask the client to use her fingers.　　　　　_____

50. Eyeliners are usually:
    a) powders　　　　　　　c) pencils
    b) creams　　　　　　　 d) cakes　　　　　_____

51. If you are holding the client's head when applying makeup:
    a) You should make sure you hold the head firmly.
    b) You should keep the head tilted back.
    c) You should hold her neck, too.
    d) You are using too heavy a touch.　　　　　_____

52. The correct order of steps in a makeup application is:
    a) consultation, exfoliation, foundation, powder
    b) consultation, moisturizer exfoliation, foundation
    c) toner, exfoliation, powder, foundation
    d) consultation, foundation, powder, concealer　　　　　_____

53. Apply blush:
    a) just above the cheekbones
    b) on the cheekbones
    c) just below the cheekbones
    d) on the apple of the cheek　　　　　_____

54. The iris is:
    a) the arch of the eyebrow
    b) the white of the eye
    c) the lower inner eyelid
    d) the colored middle part of the eye　　　　　_____

55. Bringing the eyeliner line closer to the nose:
    a) makes eyes appear closer together
    b) makes eyes appear farther apart
    c) makes eyes appear wider
    d) makes eyes appear brighter　　　　　_____

56. When applying lipliner:
    a) Have clients stretch their lips first.
    b) Have clients stretch their lips after.
    c) Hold the client's cheek with your hand.
    d) Stretch the client's lips with your fingers.　　　　　_____

57. When applying makeup for a special occasion, always:
    a) Go for a bold, shimmery effect. c) Intensify all features.
    b) Choose matte colors.   d) Consider lighting first. _____

58. For dramatic smoky eyes:
    a) Encircle eyes with a clear line of dark gray, brown, or black eyeliner.
    b) Encircle eyes with a smudged line of dark gray, brown, or
       black eyeliner.
    c) Encircle eyes with a clear line of blue, blue-green, or
       violet eyeliner.
    d) Encircle eyes with a smudged line of blue, blue-green,
       or violet eyeliner. _____

59. When applying special occasion makeup for cheeks:
    a) Use a lighter color under the cheekbones.
    b) Use a lighter color on the apples of the cheek.
    c) Use a darker color on the apples of the cheek.
    d) Use shimmer or glitter under the cheekbone. _____

60. Makeup for photographs has some special features which include:
    a) lighter amounts of product   c) heavier amounts of color
    b) lighter amounts of color   d) glossier colors _____

61. When recommending cosmetics to your client:
    a) Speak generally about color and use.
    b) Speak specifically about color and use.
    c) Concentrate on her budget.
    d) Tell her whatever is most flattering. _____

62. The two types of artificial eyelashes are:
    a) natural and artificial   c) adhesive and permanent
    b) primary and secondary   d) band and individual _____

63. Before applying artificial eyelashes:
    a) Ask the client if she is allergic to adhesive.
    b) Apply a drop of adhesive to the inner lid.
    c) Finish applying all eye color.
    d) Apply a face cloth or cotton pad saturated with warm
       water to the eye area) _____

64. Band lashes can be made of:
    a) flax   c) animal hair
    b) cashmere   d) metal filaments _____

65. The correct order of steps in applying band lashes is:
    a) Brush the client's eyelashes, curl if needed, trim the outside edge of band lash if needed, feather lash.
    b) Brush the client's eyelashes, feather band lash, trim outside edge of band lash if needed, curl if needed.
    c) Curl the client's lashes, brush client's lashes, trim the outside edge of band lash if needed, feather lash.
    d) Brush the client's eyelashes, curl if needed, feather band lash, trim outside edge of band lash if needed. _____

66. Lower lash application:
    a) is possible only with individual artificial eyelashes
    b) is impossible
    c) must be performed if upper lashes are applied
    d) is optional if upper lashes are applied _____

67. The correct order of steps when cleaning up after eyelash application is:
    a) Discard all implements, sanitize your workstation, wash your hands with soap and water.
    b) Discard disposable items, disinfect implements, sanitize your workstation, place all linens in a hamper.
    c) Discard disposable items, place all linens in a hamper, sanitize your workstation, wash your hands with soap and water.
    d) Disinfect disposable implements, place linens in a hamper, sanitize your workstation, wash your hands with soap and water._____

68. The correct order of steps in removing band lashes is:
    a) Soften adhesive with saturated pad or cloth, use cotton tips to remove any makeup and adhesive, remove the lashes.
    b) Soften adhesive with saturated pad or cloth, remove the lashes, use cotton tips to remove any makeup and adhesive.
    c) Use cotton tips to remove any makeup and adhesive, soften adhesive with saturated pad or cloth, remove the lashes.
    d) Remove the lashes, soften adhesive with saturated pad or cloth, use cotton tips to remove any makeup and adhesive. _____

69. Eye tabbing is:
    a) the procedure of applying eyeliner
    b) the procedure of applying band lashes
    c) the procedure of applying individual lashes
    d) a method of removing artificial eyelashes _____

70. The word "matte" means:
    a) thin mattress
    b) dull, nonshiny
    c) shiny
    d) heavy _____

Answer Key

1—a	36—b
2—a	37—a
3—c	38—b
4—c	39—c
5—a	40—a
6—a	41—c
7—c	42—a
8—b	43—b
9—d	44—b
10—c	45—a
11—b	46—a
12—a	47—b
13—c	48—c
14—c	49—c
15—b	50—c
16—a	51—d
17—c	52—a
18—c	53—c
19—b	54—d
20—c	55—a
21—c	56—a
22—c	57—d
23—c	58—b
24—b	59—b
25—a	60—c
26—a	61—b
27—c	62—d
28—a	63—a
29—b	64—c
30—d	65—a
31—c	66—d
32—d	67—c
33—b	68—b
34—a	69—c
35—d	70—b

Chapter *19*

THE SALON/SPA BUSINESS

1. In the beauty industry today, the term "holistic" refers to the:
   a) full range of skin care products
   b) balance of mind, body, and spirit
   c) greater emphasis on profitability
   d) profusion of specialty salons   _____

2. Increasingly, spas have been integrating Eastern practices such as:
   a) seaweed wraps   c) water therapies
   b) full-body massages   d) Vichy showers   _____

3. The greatest demand for improved spa treatments comes from which age group?
   a) 25 to 34   c) 45 to 54
   b) 35 to 44   d) 55 to 64   _____

4. Increasingly, salons require an esthetician to be knowledgeable about:
   a) the latest fashions
   b) contract negotiation
   c) complex scheduling software
   d) sophisticated medical esthetic procedures   _____

5. A primary requirement for an esthetician working in a service-oriented industry is a:
   a) desire and willingness to work with people
   b) strong drive to beat out the competition
   c) stylish wardrobe
   d) good sense of humor   _____

6. An important first step in working with a client is to:
   a) inquire about possible phobias
   b) ask for payment
   c) do a skin analysis
   d) offer a refreshment   _____

7. Solid expertise, together with prompt, attentive service, is the best way to:
   a) build client confidence
   b) sell skin care products
   c) increase your salary
   d) develop a professional network   _____

8. To make a good transition from student to professional esthetician, you must:
   a) have medical clearance
   b) establish goals and high behavioral standards
   c) purchase personal malpractice insurance
   d) learn innovative techniques   _____

9. An esthetician recognizes that the needs of the salon are:
   a) less important than personal growth
   b) not as important as the client's
   c) more important than personal concerns
   d) the manager's concern   _____

10. A well-run business provides written company policies and procedural guidelines in a:
    a) charter   c) mission statement
    b) company handbook   d) business plan   _____

11. Calling in sick is a(an):
    a) option   c) privilege
    b) responsibility   d) law   _____

12. What is a company's "mission statement"?
    a) summary of philosophy and goals
    b) rules and regulations for employees
    c) definition of employee benefits
    d) financial plan   _____

13. You can learn who the key players are in your company from its:
    a) strategic business plan   c) organizational chart
    b) mission statement   d) employee manual _____

14. Why do some salons have specific standards for performing treatments in a certain way?
    a) to keep costs to a minimum
    b) to maximize efficiency
    c) to ensure quality and safety
    d) to avoid wasting supplies   _____

15. Before beginning any new procedure, be sure to determine if your client has:
    a) a payment plan
    b) contraindications or sensitivities
    c) phobias
    d) medical insurance   _____

16. To protect yourself and your employer from liability, have your client sign a:
    a) malpractice waiver   c) permission slip
    b) medical statement   d) consent form   _____

17. Should a dispute arise with a client:
    a) document the incident
    b) notify the police
    c) discontinue treatment
    d) call the owner immediately   _____

18. A smart manager expects employees to be equally:
    a) well dressed   c) compensated
    b) driven   d) invested in common goals   _____

19. To be a team player you must be:
    a) responsible and cooperative
    b) critical and demanding
    c) jovial and fun-loving
    d) aggressive and driven   _____

20. A performance evaluation is an excellent opportunity for you to:
    a) air grievances about company policies
    b) learn ways to enhance your professional growth
    c) discuss another employee's shortcomings
    d) learn more about company finances   _____

21. To achieve your goal of owning a salon, you must be:
    a) adventurous
    b) highly creative
    c) aggressive and cut-throat
    d) focused, disciplined, and driven _____

22. Booth rentals offer the practitioner an opportunity to operate a salon:
    a) at local fairs
    b) at trade shows
    c) in a health or exercise facility
    d) in shopping malls _____

23. One advantage of a booth rental is the opportunity to:
    a) try out different business locations
    b) provide walk-in spa services
    c) run a salon maintained by someone else
    d) run a business with minimal investment _____

24. Before you begin a new business, you must first have a(an):
    a) strategic business plan
    b) charter
    c) office manager
    d) client list _____

25. Before searching for a location for your new salon, you must first determine your:
    a) furniture layout
    b) decorating scheme
    c) company logo
    d) target market _____

26. Location, accessibility, and parking for your new business are crucial to:
    a) retain clientele
    b) guarantee profitability
    c) attract business
    d) control costs _____

27. When designing a logo for your salon, it is wise to:
    a) keep things simple
    b) make a loud statement
    c) be cute and trendy
    d) select bold colors _____

28. A good way to determine if a location will attract your target market is to study the area's:
    a) ethnology
    b) geriatrics
    c) petrology
    d) demographic. _____

29. Many successful business are positively motivated by:
    a) greed
    b) competition
    c) necessity
    d) animosity _____

30. To make informed decisions as you plan your salon, you must have a:
    a) casual, flexible approach
    b) clear business plan
    c) willingness to make choices as you go
    d) general idea of what to expect   _____

31. Fixed costs for your business include:
    a) bills for supplies   c) monthly income
    b) advertising expenses   d) rent and loan payments   _____

32. Advertising expenses for your business are considered:
    a) fixed costs   c) profit margin
    b) revenue stream   d) variable costs   _____

33. Above all, a good physical layout for a salon or spa offers:
    a) good traffic flow   c) comfortable furnishings
    b) a large waiting area   d) colorful artwork   _____

34. To open a salon, compliance with local, state, and federal regulations is:
    a) mandatory   c) optional
    b) recommended   d) unnecessary   _____

35. Workers' compensation insurance is provided by:
    a) local and state governments
    b) the federal government
    c) employers
    d) workers' private insurance policies   _____

36. The Occupational Safety and Health Administration (OSHA) regulates:
    a) workers' compensation benefits
    b) workplace sanitation and safety
    c) business insurance costs
    d) liability insurance claims   _____

37. The sole proprietor of a business:
    a) is responsible for all business policies and decisions
    b) rents space from a larger organization
    c) shares managerial duties but functions as a CEO
    d) heads the board of directors   _____

38. In a business partnership, two or more people:
    a) are known as a corporation
    b) must become stockholders
    c) must have equal ownership
    d) do not necessarily have equal ownership _____

39. In a corporation, three or more people become:
    a) owners of linked but separate businesses
    b) independent business owners
    c) stockholders
    d) equal partners _____

40. If you would like to own a salon but do not have the time or energy to start from scratch, a good option is to:
    a) purchase an existing salon
    b) find a partner who can do most of the work
    c) lease a space first to motivate yourself
    d) insist that family and friends help out _____

41. Specifying who is responsible for renovations and repairs is essential when:
    a) designing a salon   c) selecting a business location
    b) purchasing salon insurance   d) leasing a salon _____

42. Offering advice or making recommendations beyond your licensing boundaries:
    a) may be a violation of medical practice laws
    b) is acceptable for minor medical conditions
    c) is normal procedure for a trained esthetician
    d) increases your value to your clients _____

43. Part of being a good business manager is knowing how to:
    a) keep employees from knowing too much
    b) delegate certain responsibilities
    c) take full responsibility for every detail
    d) be authoritarian _____

44. A reliable accounting system will help you:
    a) access financial information and plan the allocation of funds
    b) create pricing based on value
    c) adjust line expenses to enhance your bottom line
    d) determine which employees are stealing supplies _____

45. Good employee and customer relations are primarily dependent upon:
    a) providing top-notch amenities
    b) good communication skills
    c) company profitability
    d) finding good employees and clients _____

46. Pricing for products and services should be based on:
    a) value   c) profit goals
    b) client income   d) employee costs _____

47. To avoid conflicts with appointment scheduling issues, a good salon:
    a) takes responsibility for frequent appointment reminders
    b) allows busy, important clients wide latitude
    c) clearly posts specific business policies
    d) recognizes that the customer is always right _____

48. Business records should follow:
    a) proper bookkeeping standards
    b) any convenient system set up by the employer
    c) an established computer program approved by the IRS
    d) a special template provided by the IRS _____

49. Payroll, financial records, and canceled checks are generally kept for:
    a) 2 to 3 years   c) 10 years
    b) 7 years   d) 20 years _____

50. Purchase and inventory control enables you to:
    a) monitor sales receipts
    b) keep track of fixed costs
    c) calculate profits
    d) prevent shortages or overstocking _____

51. The best way to track customer preferences, measure performance, and analyze marketing trends is to maintain detailed:
    a) financial records   c) client records
    b) inventory control   d) business goals _____

52. To make a good first impression on clients, the reception area of your salon should offer a sense of:
    a) intense, constant activity   c) trendy and upscale fun
    b) calm, order, and organization d) serious corporate focus _____

53. The most important responsibility of a polished, well-trained receptionist is to:
    a) assure customer satisfaction   c) answer the telephone
    b) look attractive   d) sell retail products   _____

54. To help maintain a full appointment book, it is important for the receptionist to:
    a) sell new treatments and services
    b) promote individual practitioners
    c) encourage clients to schedule appointments during off-hours
    d) encourage clients to book their next appointment   _____

55. You should return telephone calls:
    a) at the same time each day
    b) promptly
    c) whenever you have a free moment
    d) early the next day   _____

56. An employee's job description lists:
    a) specific duties and responsibilities
    b) detailed salary information
    c) guaranteed benefits
    d) bonus requirements   _____

57. Guidelines for employees about company policies are usually contained in a:
    a) strategic business plan   c) employee manual
    b) job description   d) consent form   _____

58. A good way to motivate your employees to work as a team is to:
    a) encourage competition for wages
    b) offer a variety of performance incentives
    c) compare employee productivity
    d) withhold praise for individual achievements   _____

59. The best managers are strong:
    a) team leaders   c) rule enforcers
    b) team players   d) financial wizards   _____

60. The business of developing positive relationships and a good public image is commonly referred to as:
    a) demographics   c) public relations
    b) competition   d) staff development   _____

Answer Key

1—b	31—d
2—a	32—d
3—c	33—a
4—d	34—a
5—a	35—c
6—c	36—b
7—a	37—a
8—b	38—d
9—c	39—c
10—b	40—a
11—b	41—d
12—a	42—a
13—c	43—b
14—c	44—a
15—b	45—b
16—d	46—a
17—a	47—c
18—d	48—a
19—a	49—b
20—b	50—d
21—d	51—c
22—c	52—b
23—d	53—a
24—a	54—d
25—d	55—b
26—c	56—a
27—a	57—c
28—d	58—b
29—b	59—a
30—b	60—c

Chapter *20*

SELLING PRODUCTS AND SERVICES

1. Recommending and providing clients with quality skin care products and services is:
   a) a way to increase your income
   b) a professional responsibility
   c) taking advantage of clients
   d) not the esthetician's responsibility _____

2. According to one of the basic principles of selling, which should you do?
   a) personalize your approach for each client
   b) approach all clients in the same consistent way
   c) alternate between a few general approaches
   d) customize your approach to match the salon owner's products _____

3. In order to refine your sales approach to meet client needs, what do you need to understand?
   a) the client's budget
   b) the client's motivation to purchase products
   c) your salon's sales goals
   d) emerging trends in skin care _____

4. What is meant by "upselling" services?
   a) selling more services than your competitor
   b) raising the price on services
   c) selling additional services to current clients
   d) praising a service more than it deserves _____

5. Where can you find out a manufacturer's theory behind its products and techniques?
   a) instruction booklets   c) procedural guides
   b) marketing materials   d) all of the above are correct _____

6. Which is a good way to assess the credibility of a product?
   a) test it on your client
   b) test it on yourself
   c) learn about your colleagues' experiences with the product
   d) both a and b are correct _____

7. What is the ultimate product sales test?
   a) whether your clients want or need it
   b) whether you receive a high percentage of the price
   c) whether it causes the client a rash or other discomfort
   d) whether it helps your salon meet the monthly sales goal _____

8. When is the ideal time to obtain a complete client profile and investigate the client's skin care habits?
   a) though the mail, before the first appointment
   b) over the telephone, before the first appointment
   c) just after the first appointment, either through the mail or over the telephone
   d) during the client's first appointment _____

9. What is client record keeping?
   a) the esthetician's personal notes regarding the client
   b) the client's record of home care treatments
   c) the client's record of the amount paid and on what date
   d) the salon's list of clients' outstanding payments _____

10. Which strategy is most important for retaining clients?
    a) free treatments and products
    b) marketing and advertising
    c) personal attention
    d) such extras as refreshments, valet parking _____

11. What is a common pitfall in the relationship between the esthetician and even the best customer?
    a) disagreement on the appropriate treatment
    b) failure to provide undivided attention to the client
    c) becoming complacent and failing to provide excellent service each time
    d) failing to really listen to the client _____

12. What is the first step in educating clients about their options?
    a) explaining how you like to work
    b) understanding what the client wants
    c) promoting your favorite treatments and products
    d) discouraging them from expecting too much too soon _____

13. Which is the best time to give the client long explanations about products or treatments?
    a) during the closing consultation
    b) over the telephone after the first appointment
    c) in a detailed mailing before the first appointment
    d) long explanations confuse the client and should be avoided _____

14. Which is the correct order for the first three steps in marketing?
    a) identify the product, identify the product's benefits to the consumer, develop a complete marketing and advertising campaign, determine equitable price for the product
    b) identify the product, determine equitable price for the product, develop a complete marketing and advertising campaign, identify the product's benefits to the consumer
    c) identify the product, develop a complete marketing and advertising campaign, determine equitable pricing for the product, identify the product's benefits to the consumer
    d) identify the product, identify the product's benefits to the consumer, determine equitable price for the product, develop a complete marketing and advertising campaign _____

15. What does "promotion" include?
    a) advertising
    b) public relations
    c) personal selling
    d) all of the above are correct _____

16. What makes up a large percentage of a salon's revenue?
    a) retail sales
    b) tips
    c) donations
    d) renting space to estheticians _____

17. What purpose can be served by promotional items that tie into treatments?
    a) generates interest in new treatments
    b) helps dispose of old samples
    c) gives favored clients special attention they deserve
    d) helps reorganize salon's product inventory _____

18. What is the most important piece of information you should know about a publication before you place your ad in it?
    a) how long each issue of the publication is on the newsstands
    b) who reads the publication
    c) which other salons also advertise in that publication
    d) whether you can provide the publication staff with free treatments in lieu of payment _____

19. When business is slow and income is weak, you should:
    a) temporarily cancel your advertising
    b) spend about the same amount on advertising
    c) spend less money on advertising
    d) spend more money on advertising   _____

20. What can you hope to gain by performing community service?
    a) payment   c) favorable publicity
    b) tips   d) all of the above are correct   _____

21. Who ultimately controls publicity?
    a) the person seeking the publicity
    b) no one
    c) the public
    d) the media   _____

22. Which organizations may be willing to distribute your promotional literature?
    a) small business associations   c) other skin care colleagues
    b) other skin care salons   d) all of the above are correct _____

23. Which is a good, relatively inexpensive way to begin the networking process?
    a) radio advertising
    b) direct mail advertising
    c) sending simple notes with your business card
    d) mailing out flyers containing coupons   _____

24. What might you include in a brochure?
    a) the manufacturer's policies and philosophies
    b) your policies regarding bookings and payment
    c) the salon owner's annual budget
    d) lists of ingredients in products you sell   _____

25. What do the retail displays in most salons feature?
    a) one product line to avoid confusion
    b) many product lines, including those that the salon does not use
    c) several product lines that vary in price and focus
    d) none of these—most salons do not have retail displays   _____

26. Which statement regarding retail displays is true?
    a) they should change to coincide with the salon's themes or promotions
    b) they should not change; they should be consistent
    c) they should be kept out of the busy reception area
    d) most of a salon's promotion budget should be spent on retail displays _____

27. Ultimately, who must close the sale?
    a) the client
    b) the esthetician
    c) the salon owner
    d) the salon's receptionist/ sales aide _____

28. During the consultation, if a client seems overwhelmed by sophisticated ingredients and technology, what can be helpful?
    a) a prescriptive memo
    b) a more elaborate explanation
    c) repeating the instructions a few more times
    d) revising your product and treatment recommendations _____

29. How soon after the appointment should you place a follow-up phone call to a client starting a home care regimen?
    a) 24 hours
    b) one week
    c) such a call is not necessary
    d) 48 hours _____

30. How will you know when you have met with success?
    a) when you surpass your income goals
    b) when others seek your opinion
    c) when you can retire
    d) when you are able to lure clients from other salons _____

Answer Key

1—b	16—a
2—a	17—a
3—b	18—b
4—c	19—d
5—d	20—c
6—c	21—d
7—a	22—a
8—d	23—c
9—a	24—b
10—c	25—c
11—c	26—a
12—b	27—b
13—a	28—a
14—d	29—d
15—d	30—b

Chapter *21*

GOALS AND LONG-TERM PLANNING

1. The first step in making a decision to become an esthetician is:
    a) defining the reasons you think esthetics would be fulfilling
    b) defining the reasons you think clients would like you
    c) defining the kind of salon you would like to work in
    d) defining your financial desires and goals _____

2. If you have been offering facials at a day spa for two or three months and you're not enjoying your work, is it okay to change jobs?
    a) No, you should wait to see if it grows on you.
    b) No, it's important to show that you don't give up.
    c) Yes, although it's best not to change jobs too often, sometimes it's necessary to find a better fit.
    d) Yes, moving around shows new employers that you are aggressive. _____

3. If you have a job lined up after graduation, it's best to:
    a) Enjoy the end of school without thinking about employment.
    b) Become a client at your expected place of employment.
    c) Continue to take advantage of school job-hunting services so you get a global perspective of the field.
    d) Look for a better opportunity while you still have time. _____

4. Which of the following can be good resources for enhancing your professional status?
    a) guest lecturers at your school   c) other estheticians
    b) trade publication   d) all of the above are correct _____

5. If you have been proactive about gathering information on esthetics as a profession, it is likely you'll be able to begin your first job:
   a) knowing more than your fellow employees
   b) confidently, being able to interact with your colleagues professionally
   c) without having anything else to learn
   d) knowing as much as your fellow employees _____

6. The key attributes that employers and clients will look for in your services are:
   a) artistry, aptitude, and attitude
   b) appearance, artistry, and attitude
   c) aptitude, attitude, and appearance
   d) aptitude, appearance, and artistry _____

7. To instill employer and client confidence in your ability, it is important that you:
   a) are able to respond thoughtfully to questions about skin care routines and products
   b) personally use all of the products that you recommend
   c) try out all new skin care trends and products
   d) none of the above are correct _____

8. To reassure clients that you are a competent professional, be sure to frame and hang:
   a) letters from happy clients
   b) copies of your diploma and esthetician's license
   c) before and after photos of some of your clients
   d) copies of your teachers' letters of recommendation _____

9. Which of the following should you keep at work?
   a) deodorant
   b) toothbrush, toothpaste, and breath freshener
   c) basic toiletries
   d) all of the above are correct _____

10. Are fantasy makeup and funky jewelry appropriate while working?
    a) Yes, they show the client that you have flare and artistry.
    b) Yes, they give the client an idea of what he or she might like to try.
    c) No, they are impractical and detract from a professional image.
    d) No, they are distracting to the client. _____

11. Which of the following is NOT a quality that employers look for as they evaluate estheticians?
    a) productive problem solving
    b) no mistakes
    c) ability to learn from criticism
    d) dependability _____

12. What is the first element of effective time management?
    a) careful planning
    b) an accurate watch
    c) a thorough and accurate appointment calendar
    d) speed in completing services _____

13. If you clean and prepare your workstation at the end of each workday you are likely to:
    a) have the psychological advantage of feeling prepared to face the new day's challenges
    b) be less stressed if you run into uncontrollable delays such as traffic jams
    c) be calm and relaxed when your first client arrives on the new workday
    d) all of the above are correct _____

14. Your licensing test is coming up soon. Which of the following will you do to make sure you're prepared?
    a) Review the tests and quizzes you've already taken.
    b) Compare other states' licensing tests with the one you'll be taking.
    c) Scan the content of your textbooks to see how vocabulary words are used in sentences.
    d) Clear your calendar so you can cram the week before the test. _____

15. A licensing test should be viewed as a positive opportunity because:
    a) It is the key to achieving a goal for which you've worked hard.
    b) It's a chance to find out what you don't understand before offering your services to clients.
    c) It's a chance to find out what you don't understand before offering your services to employers.
    d) It's a chance to prove to yourself that you have learned the things you need to know. _____

16. Which of the following words generally indicates that the answer to a true/false question is "false?"
    a) never
    b) almost always
    c) sometimes
    d) usually _____

17. On a multiple-choice question with six options, you can eliminate one because it is not sensible, but the other five options all seem as though they might be correct. What will you do?
    a) Check to see if two answers are opposites. If so, eliminate them both.
    b) If there is no penalty for an incorrect answer, guess.
    c) Check to see if two answers are similar. If so, eliminate them both.
    d) none of the above are correct _____

18. When taking a practical exam, which of the following is critical to your success?
    a) thoroughly reviewing all notices and brochures sent to you in advance
    b) rehearsing with a teacher, a professional esthetician, a classmate, or on your own
    c) reviewing and practicing safety and sanitation steps
    d) all of the above are correct _____

19. How much time will the average prospective employer spend reviewing your resume before deciding whether or not to grant you an interview?
    a) 20 seconds
    b) 3 minutes
    c) 5 minutes
    d) the length of time it takes to read your resume completely _____

20. If you were applying for a job in a medical esthetics practice, which of the following would be the most appropriate word choice for your resume?
    a) I have a strong desire to help clients feel beautiful after they have been through trauma)
    b) I have a strong desire to help clients heal after they have been through trauma)
    c) I have a strong desire to help patients feel beautiful after they have been through trauma)
    d) I have a strong desire to help patients heal after they have been through trauma _____

21. For which of the following employers might a resume on brightly colored paper be appropriate?
    a) a chic day spa   c) a conservative salon
    b) a medi-spa   d) all of the above are correct _____

22. Which of the following is NOT appropriate in an esthetician's resume?
    a) sales ability   c) personal references
    b) licensing information d) administrative skills _____

23. When writing a resume, which of the following would be the best word choice to describe a professional position?
    a) served 15 clients per week
    b) performed facials and hair removal for 15 clients per week
    c) performed 10 facials and 10 leg waxings each week
    d) performed an average of 15 facials per week for both regular and walk-in clients   _____

24. How many resumes should a job-seeker have?
    a) one, so that any job listing can be replied to immediately
    b) two, one conservative and one with more flare
    c) two, one for beauty salons and one for medical placements
    d) as many as are necessary to target the needs of each job opportunity   _____

25. Which of the following resume job objective statements is likely to encourage an employer to respond to your resume?
    a) I am seeking a position that will allow me to excel as an esthetician, and I hope to advance to manager within two years.
    b) I am seeking a position that will allow me to excel and grow as an esthetician, and I hope to be a key player in a client-friendly salon team.
    c) I am seeking a position that will allow me to excel and grow as an esthetician. My long-term goal is to own and run a salon.
    d) I am seeking a position that will allow me to hold a lot of responsibility, and I hope to be a key player in a client-friendly salon team.   _____

26. To begin the resume writing process:
    a) gather diplomas, licenses, and other career related paperwork
    b) make a list of the qualifications outlined in a job ad
    c) write your career objective
    d) outline your previous jobs   _____

27. Which of the following can be hand-written rather than typed?
    a) If you don't have access to a computer, your cover letter, resume, and thank you note can be hand-written.
    b) Your cover letter and thank you note can be hand-written, but a resume must be typed.
    c) Your cover letter, resume, and thank you note must all be typewritten to show that you are a professional.
    d) Your cover letter and resume must be typed, but a hand-written thank you note is appropriate and can be more personal.   _____

28. What should be included in a cover letter?
    a) a description of the position for which you're applying
    b) an explanation of the reasons you think the particular employer could benefit from your particular background and experience
    c) a brief explanation of the reasons you work as an esthetician
    d) all of the above are correct   _____

29. Salary requirements should not be mentioned in a resume or cover letter. When can you break this rule?
    a) when you are applying to a particular salon specifically because you know it pays well
    b) when you have a minimum salary you can accept because you must repay your professional school loans
    c) when a listing in a newspaper or on an online job board says to include salary requirements in your cover letter
    d) all of the above are correct   _____

30. If you have a portfolio of your work, when should you present it to a prospective employer?
    a) Send it with your resume to give you an advantage over other applicants.
    b) Bring it with you to your interview and ask the employer if he or she would like to see it.
    c) Open it and show it to the employer as the interview begins.
    d) Wait until the employer asks if you have a portfolio.   _____

31. What is the most important consideration in choosing a prospective employer?
    a) What is most important to one person might not be i mportant to another.
    b) Salary is always most important because a high salary indicates that the company will remain profitable.
    c) Ethical considerations are most important; an ethical employer guarantees that you will be treated well.
    d) Opportunities for advancement should take precedence over other considerations. A dead-end job is guaranteed to make you unhappy.   _____

32. What is likely to happen if you are not honest with yourself or your employer about your hours of availability?
    a) You'll perform poorly, and your clients won't get the service they deserve.
    b) You're employer will find you to be undependable and your job could be threatened.
    c) You'll perform poorly and will feel stressed and unfulfilled.
    d) all of the above are correct   _____

33. Should you consider a company's cultural or political philosophy before you agree to work for them?
    a) No, cultural and political issues don't affect a workplace.
    b) No, cultural and political issues shouldn't be discussed or considered in a workplace.
    c) Yes, if you hold passionate beliefs about issues that might come up on the job.
    d) Yes, even if you feel you're not affected by others beliefs, most companies expect employees to have strong ideals.   _____

34. One of the reasons you became interested in becoming an esthetician was that you always felt great after treatment at a certain salon. You know they have no job openings, what should you do?
    a) Try to work somewhere else to increase your skills, and call when you know there is an opening.
    b) Call to ask for an informational interview to begin to build a relationship.
    c) Wait to start working until they have an opening. You don't want to be obligated to someone else when a position opens up.
    d) Call some of their clients and ask them to recommend you to the owner as an additional employee.   _____

35. Which of the following would be an appropriate way to begin a phone request for an interview?
    a) Hello, my name is Jane Doe, and I'm a student at the Glade Institute for Beauty Science, do you have a moment?
    b) Hello, I'm a student at the Glade Institute for Beauty Science, do you have a moment?
    c) Hello, my name is Jane Doe, and I'm a student at the Glade Institute for Beauty Science, may I speak to the person who hires people?
    d) Hello, my name is Jane Doe, and I'm interested in finding out more about working as an esthetician, would you be willing to speak with me?   _____

36. Which of the following is NOT an appropriate question for an informational interview?
    a) Are estheticians responsible for additional product sales?
    b) What kinds of customer service skills do you like an esthetician to have?
    c) If I were to get a job here in the future, are the salary and benefits good?
    d) How do you build your client list?   _____

37. What kind of salon is likely to offer services that promote healthy aging?
    a) independent skin care clinic
    b) medi-spa
    c) full-service salon
    d) wellness center _____

38. If you're a person who loves both meeting new people and encouraging clients to take new chances, you're likely to be very happy at a:
    a) spa in a hotel or resort
    b) chic day spa
    c) wellness center
    d) medical spa _____

39. When you go on a job interview you should:
    a) Keep makeup simple, and wear a neutral-colored suit; make a statement about your personal taste with your jewelry.
    b) Keep makeup and jewelry simple, and wear a neutral-colored suit.
    c) Your appearance is part of your portfolio; wear makeup, jewelry, and clothing that demonstrate your artistic flare.
    d) Keep makeup and jewelry simple, and wear neutral-colored selections of the latest fashions to demonstrate your knowledge. _____

40. By law, prospective employers are permitted to ask questions about:
    a) drug use
    b) birth date
    c) marital status
    d) medical conditions _____

41. A good business role model for an esthetician:
    a) should be an esthetician whose work habits and character traits are worth modeling
    b) should own his or her own salon
    c) should be any professional whose work habits and character traits are worth modeling
    d) should read trade magazines and attend trade shows _____

Answer Key

1—a	22—c
2—c	23—d
3—c	24—d
4—d	25—b
5—b	26—a
6—c	27—d
7—a	28—d
8—b	29—c
9—d	30—b
10—c	31—a
11—b	32—d
12—a	33—c
13—d	34—b
14—a	35—b
15—c	36—c
16—a	37—d
17—d	38—a
18—d	39—b
19—a	40—a
20—d	41—c
21—a	